Beyond Goodbye

Beyond Goodbye

60 days of support through grief

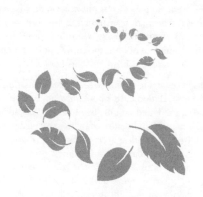

ZOË CLARK-COATES

First published in Great Britain in 2019 by Orion Spring
This paperback edition published in 2020 in by Orion Spring
an imprint of The Orion Publishing Group Ltd
Carmelite House, 50 Victoria Embankment
London EC4Y 0DZ

An Hachette UK Company

1 3 5 7 9 10 8 6 4 2

A CIP catalogue record for this book is
available from the British Library.

ISBN (Paperback) 978 1 4091 8540 6
ISBN (eBook) 978 1 4091 8541 3

Printed and bound in Great Britain by Clays Ltd, Elcograf, S.p.A

MIX
Paper from
responsible sources
FSC® C104740

www.orionbooks.co.uk

ORION
SPRING

Contents

Introduction   1
My Story in Brief   5

PART ONE   17

1. THE START OF THE JOURNEY   19

The Early Days   22
What to Expect   25
What Is Normal?   28
Common Questions   30

2. LOSING A LOVED ONE   33

Stories from those who are grieving   48

3. PRACTICAL CONSIDERATIONS   125

Fear After Losing Someone You Love   125
Intimacy (or Lack of) Post-loss   129

Returning to Work   141
Social Media   148
Special and Notable Occasions   153

4. POST-LOSS   156

Supporting the Bereaved   156
Proactive Advice for Family and Friends   172

5. LAYERS OF GRIEF   183

Healing   189
The Quest for Happiness   193
10 Questions   198
Questions I asked the Bereaved   208

PART TWO: 60 DAYS OF SUPPORT
AND JOURNALLING   215

Help and Resources   337
Thank You   339
Legacy Scheme   342
About the Author   343

Introduction

This book deals with a huge subject and I am sure many of you have opened up *Beyond Goodbye* to see what the pages might contain. My personal experience with grief means I know what it's like to feel desperate and how those feelings can make you seek out every book available to man – and woman – in the hope that it can rescue you from pain.

Let me tell you at the start: however helpful (I hope) this book may be to you on your journey, it won't save you from the agony you are experiencing if you are grieving. Oh, how I wish it could; that is what I wanted when I went looking for self-help books, and I long to be able to give you that – but nothing like that exists in the world. There is no fast pass through grief – it has to be felt and lived – so please read this book with that in mind. This isn't a lifeboat sent to drag you out of the water; it's a friend with a life ring hoping to make you feel less alone, and a guide to help you navigate the rough seas ahead.

I could have written a clinical book full of medical information and facts, of which there are many. But that is the last thing I personally would have wanted when journeying through the dark night of my soul. While I was in a fog of grief, any information I did read blindsided me with terminology I often didn't understand and facts that left me feeling cold and scared.

This made me think: what did I want? More importantly perhaps, what did I need while grieving? The answer to those questions was vital, as I knew this book needed to deliver that.

My world post-loss – after losing my babies, but also grandparents, friends and others I have loved – felt so scary and I was given very few answers, which meant I lived in a real state of uncertainty. I had hundreds of questions, and to have had just a few of these answered, or at least talked about openly, would have helped. So, I have chosen to include some topics in this book that are rarely discussed in the public domain, such as intimacy post-loss, coping with an empty house, what does good support look like?

I also needed something that helped to explain my walk through grief to others, as at the time of suffering with repeated loss I could not find the words. When you are bereft, the last thing you feel able to do is educate those around you on the grieving process, so if I'd had a book I could have given to family and friends it would have been the ultimate gift, for them and me.

I needed day-by-day support – a companion, if you like, to walk with me through grief. Following the release of my first and second books, *Saying Goodbye* and *The Baby Loss Guide*, a huge number of people told me the daily support section saved them from feeling lost and alone, so it was an easy decision to include one in *Beyond Goodbye*. I also wanted to include a journal section as part of the book, so it can become a personal diary for you. Some may fill it in and never look back at what they wrote, while others may find it comforting to revisit their walk through grief and see how far they have journeyed. I encourage you to make this space your own and to use it to creatively express your pain and your feelings, as the simple act of writing down your thoughts can help you process them.

Finally, I wanted a book that gave me hope. I have walked in that dark place, that black hole that feels lacking in love and devoid of grace. That is why, on leaving that horrid grief-filled room, I left a light on, by setting up the Mariposa Trust charity to support others. And now I want this book to be a light to those who need it. I want people to see it as their torch, and, by utilising the light it gives, I hope it will help them find a path out of the darkness. This is why I have included not just my views and experiences on loss, but also the stories of others. Grief is unique to every person; therefore, every person would describe it differently. But there are common feelings and emotions, and I hope that by hearing from many different people you will read things that resonate with you, and in turn this will make you feel less alone.

So, yes, I set myself a big task . . . Am I daunted? Of course. But if my words help you even in a small way, I will be happy. If they help you a lot, I will be overjoyed.

Often people tell me they are too afraid to read books on loss and grief, they fear they will be opening up a wound, but I assure you the wound is already there and, by facing the grief, you are simply allowing healing to take place, so don't be scared to continue reading.

Please come and find me on social media; I love to hear from readers and I want to hear your stories.

Much love
Zoë x

Instagram – @Zoeadelle
Twitter – @ClarkCoates
Facebook – @ZoeAdelleCC
Pinterest – /zoeclarkcoates/
Website – www.zoeadelle.co.uk

Grief is like a wildflower, it can erupt from the ground anywhere it chooses, when it blossoms we must be careful not to step on it. Instead we need to honour its existence and appreciate that love made it bloom.

ZOË CLARK-COATES

My Story in Brief

I have lost many people I love over the years – a best friend in a car accident, grandparents, aunts and uncles, friends . . . so there are many personal stories I could share here, but the one I have selected is losing my longed-for babies, as this is the grief that truly changed me forever.

I put off having children. I'd watched a close friend go through the horrendous experience of miscarriage and didn't know how I would personally cope with such a loss. However, once I had been married for over 11 years to my soulmate (we married young), and having set up a successful business, suddenly my biological clock started ticking. Yes, I too thought this was an urban myth – that one day you could be satisfied with no children, then the next you'd have a burning desire to reproduce – but it happened to me.

After a while, I started having symptoms that showed me I was pregnant, but very sadly it ended in a miscarriage, and my way of coping was to pretend it hadn't happened.

I didn't want to be one of those statistics which state that up to one in four pregnancies end in miscarriage, and surely if I didn't acknowledge it, it didn't really happen. I pushed all emotion down and we went into total denial. We later named this baby Cobi.

Within a couple of months, we were blessed with another pregnancy. We decided to keep it a secret from the family, and to tell them at Christmas, as we knew they would be surprised. There seems to be a presumption in society that if you are going to have children it will happen in the first three years of a relationship, and if there aren't signs of tiny pattering feet by then, the assumption is it's just not going to happen.

We went for our first scan, and we had a heart-stopping moment when the sonographer said, 'Are you sure you have your dates right, as I can't see anything?' Following our assurance that the dates were indeed correct, she suddenly announced, 'Oh, there it is', and on the screen we witnessed the miracle of life, our tiny baby, wriggling around, with its little heartbeat fluttering away. We were, of course, over the moon. She did mention that she could see a pool of blood in the womb, and warned me I should expect a little blood loss at some point, but not to worry about it at all. That evening I did get a little spotting, and if I'm honest I did panic. Any woman will tell you, if you see any signs of blood while pregnant, this fear just swells from nowhere. But by the following day the spotting had stopped, so peace returned.

A while later I caught the flu, and was bedridden for a week. Then, as quickly as it had stopped, the bleeding started again, but this time it felt different.

We found a clinic that agreed to scan me. After an age,

we were called into the scanning room, and the doctor immediately activated the all-telling machine. There, on the screen, we saw our baby for the second time – kicking away, showing no signs of distress or concern . . . what a relief!

We were due to go to a party on the Saturday evening, so, figuring that resting up might stop any further bleeding, I stayed in bed during the day, constantly doing that maternal stroke of the stomach, which somehow feels like you're comforting and caring for your child within. But when I got up that evening, I felt a sudden rush of blood, and I knew my baby had just died. I lay on the floor begging God to save her, crying out to the only One who truly controls life and death, but I knew deep down it was in vain. I knew she was destined to be born into heaven not onto earth. Mother's instinct? Who can say, but I knew her little heart was no longer beating within her or me.

We rushed to A&E where I was sadly met with little concern; I was even asked if it was an IVF baby as I was so upset. 'Why?' I asked. 'Is it not normal to cry over a naturally conceived child?' They had no answer. They didn't examine me, I was just told, 'There is nothing we can do, let nature take its course, what will be will be.' I was given an appointment for an emergency scan in a week's time and told to go home to bed.

The next day, the bleeding slowed down, and we left messages on numerous clinic answering machines begging for an appointment as soon as possible. The following morning, we got a call from a wonderful clinic telling us to come over and they would scan me. It was to be one of the longest journeys of my life.

After 40 minutes in the car, we were called from the

waiting area and into a small room. I was told to get on the bed, and the scanner was booted up. After what seemed like an eternity of silence, I finally willed up the courage to ask, 'Can you see the baby? Is it all okay?' I didn't really need to ask, my baby was still, the only movement on the screen came from my body, not hers. My question was met with the worst answer: 'Zoë, I'm sorry to say there isn't a heartbeat.' I screamed and then pleaded for a second scan, which the midwife did. She then went to get a consultant; he came in shaking his head, saying the same words, ones that would become very familiar to us over the coming months: 'I'm so sorry.' We were quickly put in a tiny room, where we sobbed, wailed, and clung to each other; we phoned our family and, on hearing the words coming out of our own mouths, the nightmare of our reality dawned on us: our baby had died, she was still here with us, but we would never hold her hand, or rock her to sleep. 'What now?' we asked.

We were told we could go the surgical route or the natural route. I chose the natural route, as the thought of going to a hospital where my baby would be just extracted from me seemed wrong; it was my baby, and I wanted to keep her with me for as long as possible.

What I wasn't prepared for was that the ordeal would go on for a week. A scan after a few days showed the baby had grown further, which is apparently totally normal, as the blood supply is still making the baby grow, but her heart remained still, no spark of life was seen . . . and, 'No, Zoë, sadly your baby hasn't miraculously come back to life. Yes, we know you had hoped it would happen.'

Was I wrong to hope this may be the case? That if I prayed non-stop, if I kept rubbing my stomach night and day, somehow her heart would just start up again. I had been told by a nurse that there was one case of it somewhere in the world once, so was I misguided to believe I could be the second?

We returned home and the days passed, long and slow. Someone asked me how I could allow a dead baby to stay inside me. 'Because it's my baby,' I said. Why anyone would presume that her death made her any less precious, or me any less loving, I'm not sure, but for some carrying a dead baby within is creepy, morbid and wrong. To me I was being her mother, keeping her safe in the place that had become her haven. I felt she was entitled to remain there until she decided to leave; it wasn't my place to suddenly evict her, and I was prepared to wait as long as needed for her to dictate the timing of our meeting.

A week to the day after her heartbeat stopped, labour started, and within 24 hours I had delivered my child, my daughter, Darcey.

For the next six weeks, my body raged with pregnancy hormones as it wrongly assumed I was still carrying a child. All day and night, sickness continued, along with the indigestion and headaches. What were once reassuring symbols of pregnancy were now horrendous reminders of what was no more. The oddest thing then started to occur, almost on a daily basis – complete strangers would randomly ask me if I had children. Each time it was like I was being thumped in the stomach. I instantly faced a dilemma: whether to protect the feelings of the person who had just asked me this very innocent question and simply say, 'No, I haven't', but, by doing so, I would be denying my child's existence; or bravely say, 'I have actually, but they died.' I tried both, and both felt wrong, and I quickly learnt I was in a lose-lose situation, and I should just do whatever felt right at the time.

I was met with lots of well-meaning statements like 'Well, at least it proves you can conceive' and 'Sometimes the womb just needs practice'. Thankfully, the less sensitive comments were in a minority, as I was blessed to have my husband – my hero – by my side, not always knowing what to say, but being wise enough to know that words often aren't needed, and that just to hold me would mostly be enough.

And then there were my parents, who sat with us and filled endless buckets with their own tears, while helping to empty ours. The rest of our family and friends were amazing, their support was tangible, and though most had no comprehension of what we were experiencing, they just made it clear to us that they were there, and that meant the world to us.

Some may think this extinguished the biological clock, but it didn't; it only increased my desire to have a baby, though the fear that I would never become a mum was overwhelming.

Two months later, I tragically lost my third baby (Bailey) via a miscarriage. We kept this to ourselves, as we felt the family had gone through enough, and they were under the impression we had only ever lost one baby, so to tell them about this loss would lead us to admitting to them, and to ourselves, that this in fact was our third child to grace the heavenly gates.

Then we got pregnant again, and following a frightening nine months, where we had fortnightly scans, we were finally handed our beautiful daughter, Esme Emilia Promise, weighing 6lb 15oz. The relief was profound, and there are no words to explain the elation of finally getting to hold and protect my tiny little girl.

We loved being parents so much; the thought of having another child was mentioned when she was one and a half, even though we had declared to all and sundry that we would be stopping at one! Nothing had prepared us for the amount of joy a little one can add to your life; there was nothing about being a mum I didn't love, so we decided to try for a brother or sister for Esme.

Naively, having given birth to a healthy, thriving child who went to full term, we believed our dealings with miscarriage and loss were in the past, and any further pregnancies would resemble that of our last one, rather than our first three. We were wrong.

We got pregnant, and all the initial scans were perfect, then on one of our appointments the scan showed our baby's heartbeat had simply stopped (again). Time went into slow motion when we were told, I literally couldn't speak. I wasn't prepared to tumble through that hidden trap door, from expectant mother to missed miscarriage, a fourth time. I misguidedly thought to lose a child when you already have one would hurt less, but I was wrong. It is different but not less.

You aren't grieving the fact that you may never be a mother to a living child (as you are already), but it hurts in lots of new ways – we were constantly asking ourselves whether this baby would have laughed in the same way as our little girl. Would they have talked in the same way? The grief was all-consuming and I felt like I had been pushed off a cliff edge with no warning. We named our baby Samuel.

In a bid to try to protect our little girl from seeing any

upset, I only allowed myself to cry in private and forced myself to keep things as normal as possible for her, but this was an Everest-type challenge, I'm not going to lie. I opted to take the medical route this time, and within days I found myself in a hospital bed, filling in paperwork, sobbing after two questions were asked by the nurse: 'Would you like a postmortem, and would you like the remains back?' Can any mother ever be prepared to answer such questions?

In medical terms, those who die *in utero* within the first 24 weeks of life are termed as 'retained products of conception', so perhaps you should expect to be asked these questions while filling in a form. I am one of millions, however, who feel not. I know that for some people these aren't babies, they are merely a group of cells, and I respect that this is their opinion, but to me and my husband it was our child, not just a potential person, but a person, and he deserved to be acknowledged as such.

We were blessed to get pregnant for a sixth time and, after telling the family around the Christmas tree on Christmas Eve, I went upstairs to find I had started to bleed. The bleeding continued for days, and when I finally managed to speak to a GP I was told I had definitely miscarried, and there was no need for a scan.

That crushing sadness overtook me again, and those who have experienced this first-hand will know you literally have to remind yourself to breathe; human functions just seem to disappear, as you feel you're free-falling over a ravine. I held onto the knowledge that to have my daughter would of course be enough, and that if we were never blessed with another child, we were one of the lucky couples who at least had the opportunity to raise one little girl.

So we painted a smile on our faces and gave our daughter an amazing Christmas.

However, by 5 January, I was feeling so ill I decided to go for a scan, in case I needed another operation, and to our surprise they could still see a baby and all looked okay. I was told that this by no means meant all would be fine, but it was a good sign, and I should book another scan in a couple of weeks. During this time my sickness increased, and by the time I went for my next scan I was sicker than I had ever been while pregnant.

The scan commenced and the doctor announced he could see two little lives on the screen. 'Yes, Zoë, you are having twins.' Cue me and Andy staring at him in shock and excitement in equal measure. He did warn us that one of the twins looked more developed than the other and that was not a good sign. With that information in mind, we were prepared (as prepared as one can ever be, that is) that we might not end this pregnancy journey with two healthy babies in our arms, but we prayed that we would.

Tragically, we did indeed go on to lose one of our precious babies, and we named her Isabella. Our other twin hung on, and we felt blessed to have one baby growing safely within, but heartbroken for the baby we lost.

What followed was a minefield of a pregnancy: I had to have my gallbladder removed, I had liver problems, placenta previa, my placenta was stuck to the old C-section scar, then the final blow came when I developed obstetric cholestasis, but our little warrior braved it all! When Bronte Jemima Hope finally appeared in all her glory in August 2011 she was declared a miracle baby, and I don't think we have stopped smiling since.

'Was it all worth it?' some may ask. Of course! 'Do you wish you had detonated your biological clock because it caused you so much pain?' Absolutely not. I have two wonderful little girls, whom I simply adore; they have made every single tear worth shedding. I'm so proud to be a mother, and I hope the trauma I have gone through makes me a better wife, mother and friend. My passion now is to raise my girls to love life and embrace every opportunity life hands to them. What I have learnt through the heartbreak is this: to me, every child matters, however far in pregnancy a person is. I also learnt a lot about grief. I was a trained counsellor before going through loss, but quickly realised all the training in the world can't teach you how first-hand experience of baby loss affects you.

I learnt that everyone is entitled to grieve differently; some may not even feel a need to shed a tear, some may sob endlessly, and both are fine. For the heartbroken, however, acknowledging the loss is essential and it's imperative to both physical health and mental well-being to grieve. Life may never be normal again when you have been to such depths of darkness, but we can move forwards, with as little scar tissue on the soul as possible, and saying goodbye was the key for me.

I will never forget the thousands of couples who are so desperate to have a child and continue to search for the solution to their recurrent losses, and those for whom the miracle of conception just doesn't happen – all the people still waiting for their miracle to arrive. Whatever losses my husband Andy and I have endured, we know we are truly, truly blessed to have two adorable girls to raise and hold.

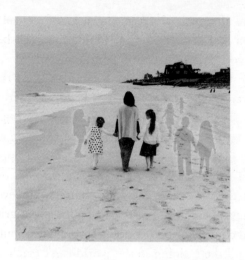

To read my story in full, please refer to my first two books, *Saying Goodbye* and *The Baby Loss Guide*.

Things don't always end up like we expect them to, or even how they were supposed to. Sometimes the worst happens, the unimaginable becomes the reality . . . But yet a strength is found to continue, whether the soul wants to or not.

ZOË CLARK-COATES

PART ONE

1

The Start of the Journey

What I would love this book to do for you is to help you see the value of grief in all of our lives, and for the words within its pages to teach you to accept its place rather than fight it – if we give grief a chair around our table, it stops it constantly knocking on our door without invitation. We need to see that grief doesn't have to be a monster living under the bed; it can be a companion we don't need to run from. When we can see pain and grief like this, it lessens the grip it has on our lives.

One of the things I have learnt on my journey is that the way we view grief and loss depends on our personal views of death and life. If we value every life, whether it be short or long, that changes how we grieve and importantly how we live. If we want to embrace life, we also need to accept death; the two go hand in hand and if we can lose the fear surrounding this often-taboo subject, we become more able to deal with the emotions that grief and loss bring.

Let me start by looking at a key question: when should someone seek face-to-face professional support when grieving?

Grief left unspoken is like shrapnel left in a wound.

ZOË CLARK-COATES

For some, professional help is needed immediately, others need it after a period of time has passed, and yet others never need it at all. Only you (and possibly your doctor) know when and if you require some additional support. There is an exception to this, and that is if you are suffering from post-traumatic stress disorder (PTSD). If you are suffering with this often-overlooked condition, you do need professional medical help. All the books in the world won't help you navigate this clinical condition, so if you have any PTSD symptoms please talk to your GP immediately. The quicker you get help, the better and more effective treatment can be, so delaying treatment is detrimental. Once PTSD is being treated, you will be able to effectively process your grief.

If at any point you feel hopeless or suicidal, please seek professional help without delay. People are not weak if they admit they need help; in fact, they are the strongest people of all.

This is my general checklist to gauge whether people need professional face-to-face support, and a 'yes' answer to any of these questions would mean I encourage them to seek help (from a doctor, nurse, grief counsellor or clinical therapist):

- Do you feel stuck in grief and are unable to move forwards?
- Do you feel the waves of grief are getting worse over time?
- Are you reliving the trauma on a regular basis?
- Are you feeling desperate?
- Do you feel vacant and removed from the world?
- Are you struggling to return to work?
- Are you unable to socialise or mix with friends or family (feeling this initially is normal, but after some time a person should be happy to re-engage with the outside world)?
- Are you avoiding things and feeling unable to face them?
- Are you struggling to eat or sleep?
- Are you relying on alcohol or other substances to help you survive?
- Are you suffering from panic attacks or anxiety that you are finding difficult or impossible to control?

The epicentre of grief is perhaps one of the scariest places on earth to reside.

ZOË CLARK-COATES

THE EARLY DAYS

The early stages of loss are merciless, and to portray it as anything other than that would be unfair and untrue. The feelings are all-consuming and overpowering. They blind-side you and can make you want to die, that is the bottom line. It is scary and unsettling and nothing can prepare you for it, but knowing it's 'normal' to feel these things helps, because when you are the one experiencing them you feel like you are going mad. So, let me reassure you, if you are feeling all these things right now, you aren't mad – you are heartbroken.

The initial days often go one of two ways. Either people switch to autopilot and just automatically do all the things that need to be done. They call people to inform them of the news, they make meals, they go through their check-list and carry out each task as if they are on a military assignment – this is the brain's way of surviving the initial trauma, and shock is helping them to carry on. It's a basic human response that most are born with, a fight-or-flight response to trauma: if someone is about to attack us, we run, we get to a place of safety before we allow our brains to process what has just happened.

Or some people shut down. They aren't even able to do basic tasks, as their brain has just pulled the plug and said nope, I just can't go there – it is like a PC on an automatic shutdown. This can happen just for a few hours, but for some it's a few days. If it's longer than a few days, I would always advise the person to seek professional help.

Once the initial shock dissipates, the 'missing them' kicks in. This void that they left in the world becomes a great big massive hole right in front of you, and you can do very little but stare at it. This is when the brain has realised the person is gone forever and it has to come to terms with their absence. Even if you were expecting the loss and felt prepared for it, nothing can actually help your brain deal with this period of time. I always say it is like a trap door has appeared and you suddenly fall. Life is okay one second, and totally changed the next. Every morning after my own losses, I would wake up and be hit with a fresh new wave of grief. There was no escape – every time a wave went over my head, it was like hearing the news that they had died all over again. It felt like I had been run over by a huge truck in a hit-and-run accident, but the lorry just kept coming back and hitting me again and again. Each time it would fling me into the air, and I would pray that was the last time it would make contact, but no, it would find me wherever I hid and hit me from a different angle.

The next stage after losing a loved one is often characterised by leaving us feeling out of control, and a natural reaction is to try to take back control of things as much as possible: doing household chores, for example, or planning events (like the funeral), undertaking work projects, or any other activities which provide distraction. It's the brain's way of trying to restore order. As it can't control the grief cycle and the feelings that surface without warning, it encourages you to take control of other things, which are probably completely unrelated to the loss, and at times can seem highly irrational to those surrounding the bereaved person. If you have any leanings to having obsessive compulsive disorder (OCD), this stage can be magnified.

It is so easy to resent your body, to fall into a trap of feeling like its failed you, it's failed your baby, it's failed your partner. Perhaps society perpetuates this by stating things like . . .' just relax and it will be okay', (which tells you your stress is making your body falter) . . . So many commonly banded about remarks, which fuel the fire of discontent and body hatred. Maybe following loss you have given up looking after yourself? Little thoughts of why bother eating right, keeping fit, or getting adequate rest . . . it is so easy to self-punish oneself, to externally manifest the internal battle of the mind that you aren't worthy of better care. I beg of you to stop listening to this negative, destructive dialogue, and to listen to the truth. You are special. Your body, however broken it may feel (and even be), deserves to be honoured, for its doing the best it can. It has earned the right to be fed, to be rested, to be nurtured and protected. Your heart has continued to beat even though its lay shattered on the floor. Your lungs have continued to inflate when you have screamed through the night. Your body, your precious, sacred body is an unsung hero, which is worthy of love.

ZOË CLARK-COATES

WHAT TO EXPECT

Here are the emotional reactions that are widely recognised as symptoms of grief:

- Shock
- Worry
- Anger
- Guilt
- Regret
- Confusion
- Relief
- Disbelief
- Denial
- Sadness
- Upset
- Acceptance

I am sure you can list even more. Grief is a like a roller-coaster and a person can experience many different emotions and feelings in a 30-minute period, and this is what adds to that feeling of being out of control – you literally have no clue how you may feel from one minute to the next.

There are also many physical reactions, as grieving is a body, mind and spirit experience. Here are some common responses:

- Headaches
- Issues with sleeping – either too much or not enough

- Lack of appetite (or at times an increased appetite depending on your relationship with food)
- Nausea
- Stomach cramps
- Upset stomach (diarrhoea or constipation)
- Lack of interest in sex or physical affection (or at times an increased desire depending on your relationship with sexual intimacy)
- Outbursts of anger or frustration
- Restless legs or numbness
- Racing heart or feelings of panic
- Nightmares
- Teeth or jaw issues (due to grinding of teeth or clenching your jaw)
- Hormonal disturbances (for example, your period)
- Depression (which is different from grieving)
- Low immunity (which can mean you catch more colds and viruses)
- Dehydration – due to crying a lot and not replacing fluids
- Hypochondria – suddenly worrying about your own health

If you are concerned about any symptoms you are experiencing, please consult your doctor. While many physical symptoms can be linked to grief, it is very important to make sure there aren't other underlying medical conditions that are being overlooked, so please don't just assume that anything you are experiencing is connected to your loss; visit your doctor to be on the safe side.

Tips post-funeral

Have things planned for the days that follow the funeral. Allow friends or family to visit, for instance. Often people have a big dip in emotion after the funeral: they tend to be on autopilot while they have an event to occupy them, but once it is over what do they focus on next? Some people go away for a few days, others don't want to stray far from home (as they often feel more secure in their home environment), but it helps to have plans for the 5–7 days after the funeral – even if it's just having coffee with a friend each day. (Any family and friends who are reading this, please be aware of this post-funeral dip and rally around. So much support vanishes after this event, and it's often when people need it the most.)

I never knew you could get annoyed with yourself for crying again, for losing it again, when you planned to be composed and all together. But that's the reality of loss, we become impatient with ourselves. We want to heal faster. We want to recover instantly, and the biggest lesson we need to learn is that we need to be kinder to ourselves. We should treat ourselves like we would treat our best friend.

ZOË CLARK-COATES

WHAT IS NORMAL?

Often people worry about what is normal, so let me re-assure you that the following are common when grieving:

- Lacking motivation
- Feeling tired
- Inability to concentrate
- Inability to make decisions (sometimes even the most basic everyday decisions)
- Inability to remember even basic information and facts
- Feeling lost and like you aren't in your own body
- Lack of identity and struggling to remember who you are
- Unhappy or unsettled in your job (and questioning your career path)
- Uncertainty about key relationships and questioning how happy/satisfied you are with them
- Insecure about things you need to do
- Unstable emotionally
- Craving to be alone
- Craving to be with people and not alone (possibly being scared of being alone)
- Fearing the future
- Feeling impatient and having a much lower anger or irritational threshold
- Intolerant of things that never previously bothered you
- Feeling the world is unjust and unfair
- Fearful of carrying out normal tasks
- Fearful of death or losing other loved ones

- Fearing something going wrong with yourself physically or mentally
- A desire to pack up and travel the world

Pain, loss and grief taught me everything I could ever want or need to know.

It taught me how to love wholeheartedly.

It taught me to embrace the now, delight in the future and celebrate the past however painful it may have been.

It was the teacher I never wanted to have, the wisest guru I had hoped to avoid.

When it entered my life, however, I had no choice but to embrace it, and my life is now better having succumbed to the lessons it taught me.

ZOË CLARK-COATES

COMMON QUESTIONS

When will these feelings end?

I know only too well why people want to know this, or how long the grieving process will take. I would have paid big money to find out the answer myself, but as grief is unique to every single person, there is no set answer. While this can be incredibly frustrating and also scary (as we all want to know the rollercoaster will end sometime soon), it can also be encouraging. 'How can it be in any way encouraging or helpful?' I hear you ask . . .

Well, we all know people who are stuck in grief and have never moved forwards, and when we are going through grief ourselves, we look at these people with eyes of terror, thinking that this is how we will now be forever. But I can confidently say to you today, that's not how it will be if you don't want it to be – that is their walk through grief, not yours. You control your walk and you can heal; you can come out of the dark part of grief, and I hope this book shows you that.

What can truly help is to forget everything you have ever been taught or told about grief – for example, that the worst part of grief is the first week – because most of what we have been taught is sadly crap. The false expectation that we put on ourselves, or others have put on us, becomes the block which we stumble over, so remove it – throw it away. You will grieve for as long as you need to grieve and not a day less than that!

Should I ask my doctor for medication?

I am not a GP and won't even attempt to tackle this subject in my book. Some people need tablets to stabilise their emotions before grief can even start to be processed, while for others medication would prevent them from processing their grief. If you feel you need medication to help you (whether that be antidepressants or sleeping tablets), talk to your doctor. Your GP can and will help you. Please also be aware that if you have any past history of depression or any other mental-health conditions, grief can act as a trigger, so chat to your doctor as quickly as possible after suffering a bereavement.

When does the 'missing them' end?

To be honest, I don't think the missing them ever ends, but in my own experience it did get easier to live with. Once the shock had passed and life became 'normal' again, those feelings just sat comfortably alongside everyday life, and I built my life around that hole, which can never be filled in. I think you adjust to it, as you don't want it filled in. Death made that hole appear, but love actually created it. It was only because you loved the person you have lost that the hole is that big and that deep, and that meaningful.

Grief is hard work, but if you can understand the process it is less overwhelming. By learning about the patterns and associated symptoms, you can get to a point where you feel as if you are controlling it, rather than the other way round, as you are able to pre-empt potential waves and, when they do hit, you can be somewhat prepared.

I encourage you to be an active participant in processing your grief, and not just become a sitting duck. The more you consciously face the pain and the trauma of loss and grief, the quicker you will emerge from the blackest part of the grieving process. It is not going to be easy, or pretty – in fact, it is going to be the hardest battle of your life, and a billion tears may need to be shed – but you will survive it.

We aren't supposed to know what to do,
we are meant to feel our way in the darkness.
As we explore, we discover that beauty lays in the
hidden locations, in the unexpected rooms,
in the places we would have never entered
if we hadn't been lost in the first place.

ZOË CLARK-COATES

2
Losing a Loved One

There are many different types of loss and each one brings with it millions of different emotions and obstacles. So while to an outsider the grief of someone who has lost a child may look pretty similar to someone who has lost their partner, for instance, the challenges will be dramatically different.

I hope by reading the many varied stories of loss in this chapter, you will feel less alone in your own walk through loss.

There are seasons when we break, and times
when we heal. There are valleys that destroy us,
and mountains that build us. The secret to surviving?
Simple! Know that there is no secret . . . There is no
fast pass and no secret tunnel to escape the pain.
You just have to face it, breathe it, weep through it,
and then one day you look up and realise the
sun has risen when you thought it would
be dark forever.

ZOË CLARK-COATES

The Loss of My Grandparents

How my grandparents came to be together is a very romantic story.

A long time ago, there were two ladies who became friends while waiting for appointments at their local doctor's surgery. Both were expecting babies, and they just hit it off . . . You know – when two people meet and suddenly you become friends for life, this is what happened to them. Funnily enough, both were called Alice.

As their bumps grew, their friendship also developed, and soon Alice McHale gave birth to a little boy called Raymond, and Alice Benbow gave birth to a beautiful girl called Florence.

A few years passed, and many happy times were spent when the two Alices got together to chat, and the children played together.

Sadly, tragedy struck, when Alice McHale became sick

and died of sepsis, leaving her husband in charge of Raymond. Adoption must have been considered, because when Alice Benbow heard the heart-breaking news, she went to the family and asked if she could adopt her dear friend's child, as she would love him as her own.

Instead of taking Alice up on this wonderful offer, the family rallied, and Raymond's grandmother and aunt pledged to help, so this little boy was able to stay in his family.

Many years passed . . . A dance was taking place. You can just picture it in your mind's eye – officers dressed up, wartime music playing. Two people caught each other's eye, and a romance developed. Soon the time came for the young lady to take this dashing young man to meet her parents.

Nervously, they entered the house, hoping that her parents would like him, so a proposal would be welcomed.

What happened next, however, no one expected!

As Raymond walked into the room, Alice looked up.

She recognised this young man. This was her best friend's little boy, the child she wanted to raise as her own. Out of all the boys, in all the world, her daughter Florence had fallen in love with Alice's boy Raymond.

Today Florence and Raymond have been married for nearly 70 years . . . and they are my amazing grandparents.

Weeks after I wrote my grandparents' romantic love story for a newspaper, my nan passed away . . . and this is the story of her loss.

Losing my nan, Florence

It was a cold but sunny March day. My nan – Florence – was dying of cancer. For weeks we had been looking after her at home following her terminal diagnosis. I don't think much in life prepares you for helping a person to die well, but the compassionate hospice nurse reassured us we could provide Nan with a comfortable departure into the next realm and fulfil her wish to take her last breath at home. So we were doing everything in our power to do just that.

Emotionally and physically it was hard. Seeing someone you love fade before your eyes, and ensuring we looked for every sign of pain when her communication skills had left her, was challenging to say the least, but we didn't want her to be in any unnecessary discomfort, so we sat watch over her 24/7.

As I look back at those weeks, a few things jump out at me. I don't view this period of my life as overly traumatic. Don't get me wrong, it was horrific in part, but it was also unbelievably beautiful. As a family we clung to each other; we laughed, we cried, we sang around Nan's bed, and we created memories that to me define what 'family' is all about.

One of the worst parts was watching my grandad break before me. He has always been so strong and dependable but his heart was breaking, and there was little we could do for him. His soulmate was vanishing, and he would often beg her to stay; the agony in his eyes still haunts me a little, if I'm honest.

As the final days drew near, we were put on constant standby, as we all wanted to be with her when she took her last breath. We took it in turns to nip to our homes and sleep and eat, and for 10 days we were regularly called with the message, 'This is it, get here fast' – and then Nan would do what she was well-known for . . . she bounced back! However, many times the doctors and nurses declared she had minutes left, Nan defied them and just kept on going. Then one night, when everyone but my mum had left the bedroom, Nan slipped into her Heavenly home, and just like that she was gone.

Seeing Nan so still was shocking. For weeks we had been watching her shallow breathing, and for that to no longer be there was hard to accept. I asked the medical team to check her thoroughly three times, as I was terrified they would take her away and she would still be alive. They patiently checked her over and over. Once her death was confirmed, all we could then do was wait for the undertaker to arrive.

Grandad sat sobbing in the sitting room. Mum had gone to bed, and all you could hear was sobbing from under her duvet.

Then my phone rang. I went to a quiet room and answered the call as I didn't know who it was. It was a call from Number 10 to tell me Andy and I had won the Prime Minister's 'Points of Light' award for all our charity work. This news should have been a lovely moment, one to celebrate, but the timing was just surreal. Receiving the call, in those moments where time seemed to stand still, felt like a gift from Nan, but as the tears flowed I was just sad she hadn't been with us to hear the news.

The undertakers then knocked on the door; two kind and patient gentlemen entered the house. They told me what they needed to do. My grandad – Ray – said he wanted someone to be with my nan at all times, but he insisted that he could not face being in the room. My sister felt she couldn't either, and my mum said there was no way she could handle it . . . so that left me! I didn't feel I could cope either, to be honest, but there was no one else there, so I said I would stay in the room.

Cards on the table here: this was one of the most traumatic moments of it all for me.

I wanted to scream, cry and beg them not to move my lovely nan. I wanted to remember her playing with us, laughing with us, not being put into a body bag.

The experience of loss is so complex, so painful and so very tough to get through, but having a family to share these moments with helps you survive it.

I was once afraid of death, of dying, but I guess I have learnt there is nothing to fear; the pain lies in leaving behind those we love, but if we know we are leaving them in a good place, surrounded by people who love them, we can be assured they will not only survive, but thrive following our passing.

My grandfather's grief was profound and all-consuming. Watching him struggle was beyond painful. On the evening of Nan's death he went missing, and we had no clue where he'd gone. We later found out that he had driven to the undertaker's and just sat outside, so he could be close to Nan, as he could not comprehend spending a night without her in his room. Even writing this makes me weep. As a family we wanted to rescue him; of course, we couldn't. All we could do was be there for him, to grieve alongside him and reassure him that Nan would always be part of our family.

For the first few years Grandad seemed to be waiting to die himself; he had lost the will to live and just wanted to be in Heaven with my nan. It was incredibly hard as a family to witness this, and even harder for him to live through the relentless grief. Then one afternoon he decided, following in the rest of the family's footsteps, to do some charity work. He called a local organisation, Westbank, that provided support to the elderly and sick, and asked if he could help them. They said yes, and the rest, as they say, is history. To date, he has helped over 50 people in the community. To say we are proud of him is an understatement.

I asked my grandfather a few questions four years after Nan's death:

What do you wish you had known prior to losing Nan?

'How great the loss would be and how overwhelming the shock would be.'

Could anything have helped you in those early days?

'No, I just needed permission to express the pain.'

How is the grief different four years on?

'The grief is still as strong even now; most things trigger memories. But I would still rather have the tears and the pain and have the memories. If I ever hear "The Anniversary Waltz" I weep, but along with the pain of losing her, happy memories sit alongside the pain.'

What do you struggle with most now?

'The loneliness, not having that conversation – I often still talk to her as though she is here with me. When I walk in the door to silence that's a hard thing to accept – who do I now tell about my day? When I roll over in bed, I still expect to feel her by my side, I reach out to touch her and it's like I lose her all over again.'

What advice would you give to someone who is grieving?

'My three top tips would be:
1. Get involved in activities and if possible serve others. I found a new purpose in life by volunteering for a charity. I was used to being needed, and by helping others I felt useful again. It is so tempting to just lock yourself away following loss, but that just increases the feelings of isolation, so I encourage everyone to re-engage with life.
2. You can expect to feel disloyal if you smile or have fun, but let me reassure you that you aren't being. Your loved one would want you to be happy again.
3. I was filled with regret once Florrie died, and the

thoughts of what I could have done to make our lives even better still haunt me. I guess this is part of being human, but talking about these worries and fears helps me cope with them.'

Three days after sitting with my grandfather and asking him these questions, he was diagnosed with cancer himself, and three weeks to the day he passed away.

I am now continuing to write this story having lost them both . . .

It's been a few hours since I stood by his bed watching him take his last breath, and the pain is indescribable. Those around me feel numb, and I would pay big money to feel numb right now, as I feel overwhelmed with raw pain. It is hard to stand; I just want to lie on the floor and howl like a child. On the day he was diagnosed with cancer, he was told he would live for another 2–10 years, but three weeks to the day he is lying in the chapel of rest and not in his bed. I feel immense shock and anger that we have been robbed of more time with him, and so terribly sad.

I am not an envious person and rarely battle with jealousy; I mostly feel joy for other people's achievements or experiences. But one area where I can't help feeling jealous is when people are able to just get on with life while grieving, to put their feelings in a box. Is it healthy? Probably not. Should it be encouraged? Rarely. But when you are engulfed with grief you would give every penny you have to be saved from it.

Today as a family we are grieving my mum's father, a father-in-law, a grandfather, a grandfather-in-law, a great-grandfather. I'm sobbing due to my pain, crying for my children's heartache, weeping for my husband's grief, wailing for my mother's suffering.

Watching someone die is a surreal experience, everything within you wants to rescue them, but all you are permitted to do is stand by their bed and watch. At the point of death, a person changes so much physically, and that in itself is shocking. Grandad looked dramatically different in an instant. All sign of him being in pain left and his skin became smoother.

He was ready to go, but we weren't ready to let him leave, yet we knew we had no choice; it was time for him to re-join my nan.

It is now a few weeks since he died and I feel ready to write more.

Telling my girls that Grandad had died was one of the worst things I have ever needed to do as a parent. They adored their great-grandfather and I felt like I was in a movie when the words came out of my mouth, and my daughters sank to their knees crying. The temptation, as any parent will know, was to tell them it will all be okay, to urge them to stop weeping, but I knew that would be doing them a disservice, so instead I told them to cry for as long as they needed to. Bronte screamed, with her head in her hands, and she quietly uttered, 'Mummy, my heart is broken forever.' I wanted to reply, 'No, it won't be, my darling,' but how could I say that? It may be changed forever, and actually that is okay – everything in life changes us, and we should not be encouraged to remain the same. So instead I said to her, 'Yes, Bronte, you will now be different, but I promise you this, you will smile again. But for now you cry as much as you want, and as hard as you want. Mummy and Daddy are here with you.'

Esme cried quietly, and just wanted to be hugged as silent tears ran down her face.

The first 24 hours were really tough for them emotionally, but within 48 hours they had amazingly accepted he had gone, and, while they still had periods of intense grief when they would sob uncontrollably, they would quickly resurface and want to play a game or go to the park.

Children and grief – my tips:

Keep reassuring them it's okay to cry, scream, beat the floor with their hands – I know you will desperately want to rescue them and you would give the world to remove their pain, but unfortunately you can't, and the best gift you can give them is to grant them full permission to process their pain and grief in whatever way they wish.

Most children will come in and out of the grief – one minute they will be beside themselves with emotion and the next laughing at something on TV; this is their way to survive it. My best piece of advice is not to discourage crying. It's so tempting to say, 'Come on, now, stop crying' or 'Let's just look at the positives that have come from the loss (e.g. no more pain)', but we can then be robbing them of the chance to deal with the loss and process the grief. The human spirit was created to grieve and mourn the loss of a loved one; this is 100 per cent natural and essential to wholehearted living. What we teach our children now sets them up for a good life that is emotionally well balanced – so it's okay to say, 'It hurts like hell right now, and the pain is crushing, but soon it won't feel like this. We will always miss them, but the raw, blackest part of grief does eventually pass, so give in to the pain, and let the tears come whenever they surface, as the tears are part of the healing.'

We have now planned my grandfather's funeral, and we are preparing to say our formal goodbyes next week. It feels really important that we make his send-off beautiful and something he would be proud of.

Post funeral – So how am I now? Well, it still seems unreal that he has gone, and the grief is immense. I do have times when I can surface and focus on work, but then the grief waves hit, and I tread water until I have the strength to swim. Grief is a journey, and I am okay with hurting. And I am completely fine with shedding public tears, because after all grief is just love with nowhere to go.

Today we are burying Grandad's ashes. It feels like the last major thing to do before he is properly laid to rest. Part of me didn't want to say anything on social media about what the day installed for me, but I also felt a need to encourage others who are walking a similar path at the moment. Whilst I was sitting at Grandad's bedside my sister took a photo on her phone of me sitting and chatting with him. Whilst this photo is pretty agonising to look at, it is now one of my favourite ever pictures, as it tells a story . . . a story of love. Here is the photo and the post I shared on Instagram.

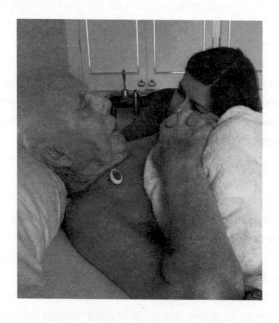

I didn't know if I would ever share this photo as it feels so incredibly personal and intimate, but it's also one of my most loved pictures. As you can see from my huge swollen eyes I had been crying endlessly for days when this picture was taken, we had sat by Grandad's bedside both day and night, listening to him chat, responding to his needs, and heartbreakingly waiting for his time to leave this earth and be reunited with Nan. I was terrified of watching him die, but I was more terrified of him dying alone. I was petrified of seeing him suffer, but more petrified of him suffering without a hand to grip onto. I could hardly cope with waiting for him to take his last breath, and would often leave the room to silently scream in the bathroom.

Sometimes fear tries to keep us out of the room. It tells us we should be scared of what we may witness, or fear saying the wrong thing. It tells us to put our own needs before another and encourages us to run, rather than telling us we have the strength to show up.

It's hard watching someone die, whether it be an adult or a child . . . but I promise you we all have the strength to be present, as love carries us through these heart-breaking moments.

So why is this picture so special to me? Well I guess it's because to me it shows pure love. It proves I showed up even though it hurt like hell. It shows how much I loved Grandad and how much he loved me. Perhaps most importantly it shows I was there till his last breath.

Grandad passed away within 24 hours of this photo being taken, but he was still chatting here and making us all laugh.

Today we bury Grandad's ashes alongside my nan's . . . though we believe their spirits are already reunited in Heaven, their bodies will today be reunited on earth.

Love you forever, Grandad, and thank you for everything ❤

It was a hard post to write, but it was also cathartic, and the response was overwhelming. People messaged me to tell me it gave them strength to now show up. People shared how they had lost grandparents in the past 48 hours and this post meant the world to them . . . and hundreds of others just reached out to share their feelings. At times its worth risking stepping out, it's worth being vulnerable and sharing from the heart. I wanted the world to know how much I loved him, and I think this post did that.

The love I carry for you makes me braver,
for now I carry your sword and mine.

ZOË CLARK-COATES

It is often helpful to understand how others have navigated their path of loss, and so here I share stories of pain and hope.

Loss of a Mother

Grief caught me totally off guard, overwhelmed me beyond words; I couldn't breathe the shock was so intense. Those initial feelings did leave and day by day I was able to adjust and find a new way of life that would honour my amazing mum. Bereavement has brought me a new respect for the fragility of life, matched with a deep, heartfelt appreciation for the time we have.

My mum loved without condition and lived fully, generously and with endless energy. My last moments with her were on Filey beach, where she played with my daughters and collected stones. That night while on a cliff-top walk my mum collapsed. She died on that cliff-top and our journey of grief had to begin. For someone surrounded with so much love and support, I had never felt such intense loneliness.

The fog of grief stayed with me for a number of weeks; I functioned but that is perhaps overselling it. I was present but very much distant and detached from what I was going through. I didn't want to eat, I couldn't make decisions and I absolutely did not want to plan a funeral.

Grief for me felt intensely private, and I felt selfish for not being in step with my sister and Dad. I did not want to talk about how I felt, reflect, or look at photos, and I actively avoided anyone who wanted to offer their condolences or hug me. Unfortunately, my mum was incredibly popular, so this wasn't sustainable at all. I listened to people's stories of grief and how they felt during similar times, and I can honestly say I didn't relate to any of them, as well-intentioned as they were. Life that was so settled and balanced had become without warning so shattered and out of control, and I replayed the trauma of the day over in my mind, finding it difficult to see people around me getting on with life while my world was experiencing this irreversible damage.

For me the turning point was normality; lying down to sleep at the end of the day was a small victory. Each morning was a day further into a new reality and each day I adjusted just a little bit more. I returned to work and allowed routine to shape each day. I miss my mum every day as we were incredibly close. That powerful aching feeling hasn't lessened at all, but I now enjoy talking about her, laughing about things she said and did, and live the type of life that I know she would have enjoyed being a part of. At the time of her death I wouldn't have thought this was possible, but taking it a day at a time and surrounding myself with people who care deeply has brought me to the point of being able to celebrate Mum and be joyful that I got to be her daughter.

I longed to rewind time. To relive a previous chapter of my book, knowing this time I wouldn't take a second for granted, as I would be acutely aware the story would end without you joining me in the sequel.

ZOË CLARK-COATES

Loss of a Wife

Chris's story

I am the husband of the late Dr Kate Granger MBE and also co-founder of the #hellomynameis campaign. July 23rd 2005 is the happiest day of my life so far, as it's the day Kate and I got married . . . fast-forward 11 years and you get to the saddest day of my life – the day that my beloved Kate passed away (aged 34) following our five-year journey with cancer.

Given that Kate was diagnosed in 2011 with a terminal form of cancer, I truly believe that my grieving process almost started then, and because Kate and I were very open about death and dying it was something I outwardly appeared to be handling well. As the time progressed, we managed to tick off various items on the bucket list and really enjoyed life, making special memories that I will always treasure and these certainly helped in the grieving process post-death. In the few weeks after Kate died, I was that busy organising her funeral, organising her belongings, informing various professional bodies etc. that I didn't have time to think about the huge event that had just taken place. My employer was amazing, as they always were before Kate died, and this ongoing support really does help.

Kate used to always say that she worried about how I would cope a few months after she died as she knew initially I would keep myself busy. Grief only really kicked in about a year after Kate had passed and even now (almost three years on) I find myself emotional at either the smallest of things or just when I want to speak to her. I would find myself talking to photos of Kate and telling her how my day has gone etc., and I always do my best to make her proud and make a difference to other people.

Grief comes in many guises and there is no fixed way for how people should react when they lose a loved one. My advice is to remember the happy times, keep family and friends around you and don't be afraid to share how you are feeling.

Love may break you, but love will also heal you, this is the oxymoron of life.

ZOË CLARK-COATES

Loss of a Husband

On Valentine's Day 2006, I met the love of my life. I was 17, with big dreams of university and an illustrious journalism career, when tanned, smiling, ambitious Nathan walked in my front door and changed everything. We fell for each other, hard. After an unforgettable summer we went to our respective universities and waited four years to be together, writing letters and talking on the phone for hours – dreaming of the day when we would never have to say goodbye again. Our wedding in June 2010 was the culmination of those long years of waiting; the most beautiful, relieving day we could have imagined. We could *finally* be together – the future was ours, and intoxicating.

Nathan and I had four years of a fairy-tale marriage. We were best friends, kindred spirits, and soulmates. He was my home, my harbour, everything I ever wanted. In September 2014 we welcomed our princess, Elissa Rose, into the world. Nathan was overjoyed to be a father. He doted on our baby girl, holding her every chance he could, marvelling at each exquisite detail and expression. We were a family of three; our happiness was complete.

But on 5 October 2014, Nathan never came home from work. A lone policeman arrived instead, to tell me that Nathan had been hit head-on by a drunk driver and was killed instantly. In a single moment my entire world crashed down around me. I went from being a glowing new mother desperately in love with my husband, to a 26-year-old widow with a newborn daughter. There was no goodbye, no chance to tell Nathan everything over-flowing in my heart for him.

In those early moments shock overwhelmed me, and duty kicked in. There were people to call, and arrangements to be made. Nathan and I had been living hundreds of miles from our families. I knew immediately that I couldn't stay another day in my city without him, and by the time I finally collapsed in bed that night, sobbing silently into Nate's pillow, our bags were packed to go home the next morning.

Grief hit me like a hurricane, leaving me writhing in anguish and disbelief. I alternated between frenzied emotion, gut-wrenching sobs, panic, and numbness. I felt like the walking dead – existing day by day somehow, but unable to make sense of anything. All my hopes and dreams for the future died on that road with Nathan.

Still navigating the complications of new-motherhood, living in a room in my sister's house so far removed from the life Nathan and I had built together, I went underground. For years I chipped away at the layers of my loss. Grief, in its truest form, is a reckoning with every memory – every moment in time, every smile, every kiss, every habit and idiosyncrasy of daily life, every shared dream for the future. It is a farewell, an admission that you alone are left to shoulder these memories, carrying them with you for the rest of your life. For a long time, I teetered on the brink of total despair. I was so very tired of breathing, of waking up yet again to face another faceless day. But I was propelled forward, by the relentless passage of time and the resiliency of the human spirit.

Four and a half years later, I have found the sunrise. Elissa Rose is the light of my life. She carries so much of her daddy in her eyes and in her soul. We have a beautiful life together; we love to laugh and travel and explore new places. I am learning, day by day, to live again.

The river of tears only results due to the ocean of love I carry for you.

ZOË CLARK-COATES

Dave's story

I will never forget the day I got a phone call from Lauren at home to say that the midwife would like her to go to the hospital as she was struggling to find our little boy's heartbeat. I could tell that Lauren was absolutely terrified so I raced home as fast as I could. I told her that it was 'just the way he was lying' and 'it would be fine', 'I'm sure they have this all the time', and I genuinely felt this was the case.

All the way to the hospital and even in the waiting room I was not worried; I'm one of those people who generally thinks everything will be fine and that if you keep positive then things just have a way of working out okay or you can always fix it.

The sonographer took just minutes to say calmly, 'I'm sorry but your baby's heart has stopped.' My world stopped – this wasn't going to be okay, I couldn't fix this! I held Lauren; I feared if I let go she would break into a million pieces on the floor.

The next weeks and months were just indescribable; the pain, the tears and the questions. Why, how, what? Telling our family, finding out what was going to happen now. I don't know what I thought would happen but I had absolutely no idea that we would have to go through the birth or plan a funeral. I just wanted it to all go away! The hardest part at that point was knowing Lauren still had our baby inside her but he was not alive; it was just too much to cope with. It was days before we went into hospital but it seemed like weeks, as grief slows down time.

It has now been some years since we lost our little one. The loss has become part of who we are, and we have found giving back to charity has helped us process this pain in a positive way.

My advice to others would be to talk about the loss, and don't listen to society when it tells you to brush the pain under the carpet – face it head-on and, I promise you, life becomes easier once the shock has passed.

Grieving can make you lie. How easy it is to just
say 'I'm fine' when you are actually broken.

ZOË CLARK-COATES

Becki's story

It was the morning of 25 June, 4.31am, and my mother and brother were sat at the end of my bed waking me up. I knew instantly something was wrong. As my mum began to tell me that my dad had died, I did the only thing I could think of doing in that moment and let out a gigantic, gut-wrenching scream. I still remember that moment now, 15 years later.

I was 16 years old, had just taken my GCSEs; I had one to go and my dad, who was a teacher away on a school trip, had died of a heart attack. He was a PE teacher with no sign of anything wrong with him. It was a total shock.

The days and months that followed are a mix of a complete blur and memories that will be etched into my mind forever.

Honestly, it was a strange combination of getting on with normal life and processing the pain but also knowing that my dad was never coming home again. My dad owned a gymnastics club and I remember doing my classes the day after because it took my mind off of what had happened. And I remember consoling friends as they heard the news and processed the pain. It was a weird mix of holding it together for other people but then collapsing into a pile of tears if I thought too hard about it.

One of the things I do remember so vividly is the morning he left to go on his school trip. I remember saying to him, 'Don't leave without saying goodbye.' I was drying my hair and, turning the hairdryer off for one second, I heard the door close. I ran downstairs, out to the car, and told him he nearly left without saying goodbye. I gave him a kiss, hugged him, waved him off and told him I loved him. I'm so grateful for that final memory of him and the perfect timing of turning off my hairdryer so I didn't miss that moment.

We had the most incredible support from friends and family in the weeks and months after. But I think the thing that got me through most was just a peace in the pit of my stomach that told me that it would all be okay. Somehow, some way, we'd make it through and we'd survive. That day I realised I wouldn't have my dad walking me down the aisle, he wouldn't meet my children or my husband, but I had peace. A peace that surpasses all understanding. I didn't understand, and I don't think I ever will, but I'm thankful for that peace.

Fifteen years on and I still think about my dad almost every day. The memories feel further away and more distant. I'm not sure I can still remember his voice perfectly but I am so thankful for the 16 years I did get with him.

Not everything that comes is supposed to stay.
Our job as humans is to get our heads around this
often devastating reality.

ZOË CLARK-COATES

Sarah's story

My husband and I were travelling the world when we fell pregnant. A pregnancy test in Thailand, an early scan in Hong Kong, and then our baby came with us to Africa. At our 12-week scan in Zimbabwe, the sonographer broke the news of 'no heartbeat' as gently as possible. It felt like my heart had stopped beating too. We clung to each other and just sobbed. It's incredible how much you can love a tiny baby whose gender and personality you'll never know.

We were spun – in that dusty African street – into the admin of baby loss. The sonographer, knowing we weren't locals, drove ahead so we could follow her to the nearest GP surgery to discuss my options. I saw the world through a teary blur, as Jonny clutched my hand and the doctor suggested a pessary immediately and a procedure tomorrow. I wanted to hold onto that little body in my body a bit longer, but knew we needed to follow medical advice. We were staying with my sister on her family's chicken farm, and returned to find a power cut – not an unusual scenario – and my sister waiting expectantly for beautiful scan photos. I saw her heart break for us as we broke our news.

That night I began to bleed heavily. The doctor had told me it would 'feel like a period, nothing to worry about'. That evening – just moments after the electricity had miraculously returned – I found myself screaming, 'He lied! He lied!' in the bathroom as the gruesome reality took hold. It felt nothing like a period. And everything like a death. Amid my desolation was a flood of gratitude. We'd seen no family in nine months, and just happened to be staying with my sister when this all unfolded. We weren't on some remote Thai island. She brought us her low-battery laptop and highly prized imported Dairy Milk, and Jonny and I tucked ourselves away from the world under our mosquito net to watch *Big*.

At the local hospital the next day, I found myself acutely grateful for the NHS. Instead of a solid roof there was corrugated iron; instead of a clean gown I was given a threadbare old blanket; and instead of electricity, another power cut. I looked around at the local women in the waiting room and knew that if it was their lifelong medical reality, it could be mine for just one morning.

Our Little Adventurer is buried under a fig tree in the red African soil.

The essence of you, fragranced every part of me.

ZOË CLARK-COATES

Losing a Young Daughter

A mother and father share:

It was the day after Mother's Day, 27 March, with a week of my 15-month-old beautiful, clever little girl, Elea, just not being herself. I took her to the GP after seeing a rash on her arms.

The doctor I saw was so lovely but obviously concerned. She told us we needed to go to hospital immediately. We arrived and waited. A cannula was put in her little hand and blood was taken. She was so pale and sleepy. My husband joined me by lunchtime and by the evening we were admitted for the night. About 10 minutes later six doctors and nurses came into our room. My heart sank. 'We are so sorry but your daughter has leukaemia. We are not sure of the type yet but she needs extra fluid and a blood transfusion.' I cried with the heartache, the heartbreak. We were in shock. How could this be happening to my little girl, my longed-for baby?

After three weeks in hospital, three general anaesthetics and lots of different medicines, we finally had a diagnosis of acute myeloid leukaemia and we were off to the Royal Marsden children's ward in Sutton, where she started her first round of chemo. Nothing quite prepares you for consenting to your child being given the worst drug in the world. It makes you grow up rather quickly in that moment.

Acute myeloid leukaemia is one of the most aggressive types of leukaemia you can get; it is particularly horrible in that it can affect young children. The treatment is usually six rounds of chemotherapy, but if the first round goes well you could be into remission quickly.

Elea, our precious daughter, had possibly the worst subtype of AML, with similar characteristics of another blood disease at the same time. Her first round of chemo looked really positive and for the first time in eight weeks we were allowed to go home! It was a glorious week. Seeing friends, having her hair cut, getting her first shoes. And just being slightly normal despite being the nurse and her mummy.

We came back into hospital and to our delight we got our own room. But the news we heard was not great. The leukaemia had not gone into remission and we were now on the stem cell transplant route.

The journey in hospital was one of hope, joy and anguish. Elea had five rounds of chemo, six general anaesthetics, 25 feeding tubes inserted, numerous antibiotics and other medicines. She was an absolute trouper, who owned the corridors of the children's ward with her walker, whose smile and wave would grab everyone's attention. The nurses were outstanding and fought over who was going to look after her. Our friends where championing us with food, visits, presents, prayers, chats. But after six months in hospital and only nine nights at home the leukaemia was too strong.

At 12.30pm on Sunday, 10 September 2017 our darling daughter went to heaven while in my arms. My husband and I were broken and shocked; we would never be able to hug her, hold her hand, play with her, see her grow up.

Grief is a rollercoaster of emotions. You never know

what you'll be like from minute to minute, hour to hour. Life is truly unfair. I can remember a moment in hospital towards the end when I just knew we weren't going to have her for much longer. I couldn't stop the tears, they just kept coming.

A year has passed and I certainly can't believe it has. I feel there are days when I miss her more than ever and just want to be playing with her, doing mummy life. Life will never be the same.

Matthew's story

Elea had an occasional temperature or sniffle and one short brush with chicken pox. That was it. While friends and family with children had an almost constant stream of coughs, colds, bumps, bruises and all the rest, when social media was announcing yet another bedridden family, my wife Jennie and I couldn't help but feel very lucky that our (eventual) bedtimes were purely due to sleep rather than anything else.

Elea had been a very happy and very healthy little girl for nearly all of 15 months when we were told, in a room with a multitude of doctors and specialists standing around us, that she had a rare subclass of acute myeloid leukaemia. There were treatments, but it wasn't going to be easy and the outcome was far from certain.

So many emotions ran through my head; fear overriding every one. My own hope was that we could do this, Elea could do this. Would I be the husband and father my girls needed, now more than ever? Would I be strong enough?

What would we do if she didn't make it? I like to think that I am a positive and optimistic person, but faced with this news, a sucker punch to my heart and soul, I just didn't know if I could do it the way I wanted to do it and Elea and Jennie needed me to do it.

It's hard to be positive when facing fear head-on. My wife and I are normal people; we're not necessarily any stronger than any other man or woman; we did what we had to do in those six months – we called it 'survival mode'. We did what we could to make our little girl happy; we cherished every moment we could. I don't think we had a choice to do anything else. Our bodies and minds wouldn't let us.

Elea endured five rounds of chemo, each one more extreme than the last. Unfortunately, the treatment just wasn't enough and we entered into palliative care, staying at the hospital so we could just look after Elea without the burden of having to nurse her, as well as be her parents. This lasted just one week. We let our little girl go to heaven on a Sunday morning, cradled in her mother's arms, with me holding them both.

Our consultant had reassured us that it wasn't anything we or she had done, it was just something that happened; but it is extremely hard to rationalise an illness that came out of nowhere, with no warning. It just didn't seem fair, any of it.

The weeks following our loss did not consist of much beyond trying to hold things together, remembering to eat and drink, and planning a funeral we had never expected to plan. A massive network of friends and family helped us through this time (and continue to) and have made our devastating loss that little bit easier to bear.

I don't think anything you do in grief is necessarily right or wrong, you just react, you do. You get through each second, minute, hour as best you can and, whatever decision is made, that's it. We both have treated our loved ones unfairly, been angry for the smallest of things, gotten upset at a song on the radio, but at the core of all these missteps is our loss. It's not an excuse but more an explanation, and I believe it is getting easier, whatever that means. We have had counselling, we have family and friends helping us, but one thing we do know: it's not a journey with a fixed timeline; I don't believe it will ever be 'completed'. It is a process and burden that will always be with me, with our family. Elea will always be missed and life's milestones will be forever bittersweet, but all anyone can do is keep moving on and try not to forget the precious, golden moments of her short, beautiful life.

Even if the oceans run dry and the clouds lay at my feet
I will love you.

If the earth ceases to spin and the seasons fail to change
I will love you.

If the mountains crumble and the valleys enlarge
I will love you.

If the moon resigns from the sky and the sun turns to ash
I will love you.

ZOË CLARK-COATES

Loss of a Husband and Son

Sandra's story

In 2013 my husband and 12-year-old son died in a walking accident in the Alps, leaving me and my 15-year-old daughter. Our family was halved and we lost all the men. Although we lost two people, we were dealing with four different bereavements. I had lost a husband and a son and my daughter had lost her dad and her only sibling.

Initially, shock took over and I learnt it was my body's way of protecting me. The pain of such catastrophic and sudden loss is too much to bear all at once and so shock brings an initial sense of numbness. This allowed me to make it through the first weeks, but soon the anaesthetic effect wore off and the pain became raw. The emotion often overflowed in wailing and sobs but sometimes it was too intense to express. There was a deep sense of protest, of desperately wanting to go back to the life I once had, and also a sense of bewilderment. How could the life I once knew be torn apart in one moment? How do I live this new life?

Going to bed was tough. I didn't want to go to sleep because when I woke up and remembered what had happened, the overwhelming pain was almost too much to bear. Each morning just getting up was hard. I would force myself into the shower and afterwards would feel utterly exhausted. I don't think anything can prepare you for the exhaustion that comes with grief. For years after, I needed more sleep than usual and with the tiredness came a sense of brain fog. I forgot things all the time and couldn't think straight. The rest of the world seemed distant and out of focus.

Knowing my daughter had lost her dad and only sibling was the worst pain of all. Yet having my daughter helped me make it through. I knew I wanted her to still be able to make the most of her remaining teenage years and I had hope that this was possible. Deep down I knew, despite what had happened to us, that we could still go on to live amazing lives and so my focus became rebuilding our world.

Meeting others who had also suffered loss helped. I attended events for those widowed young and events for bereaved parents. Talking to people who had been bereaved for longer inspired hope for the future. I also read books. Understanding the process of grief helped me to bear the pain.

Although the pain of loss is still very real, my life has expanded and grown around it. My life looks nothing like I thought it would and yet it still has meaning and purpose. My husband and son are always missing and yet I have found that you can laugh again, you can have fun, and the miracle is that joy can co-exist with the pain.

I will never forget this pain, but that is okay
as I will also never forget this love.

ZOË CLARK-COATES

Loss of a Daughter

Erin was my firstborn child. My husband and I were incredibly excited when we found out I was pregnant and overjoyed when she was born. However, within 36 hours of Erin's birth we were told she had a problem with her heart. She was transferred to a hospital 60 miles from home. The next three weeks were terrifying and ultimately devastating. Erin died when she was 22 days old after spending her whole life in hospital. I'll spend the rest of my life missing her. I miss my baby Erin, who I knew from the time we had together, and I miss my older Erin who I will never get to know.

I miss many things from the first week of Erin's life. I miss watching her stretch her entire little body and wriggle around as she was waking up from a deep sleep. I miss the way she used to gulp down her milk as fast as she could and then clamp her mouth tightly shut when she had drunk enough and refuse to let the bottle pass her lips again. I miss watching her sleep – it seemed she could get comfortable in any position. I miss it when she pursed her lips in her sleep and pulled other funny faces. I miss our cuddles; I miss our cuddles so much. I miss holding her against my chest and snuggling her close. I miss stroking her soft hair and watching her sleep, her cheek squashed against my shoulder. I miss resting my cheek on the softness of her head and feeling completely at peace, knowing that this felt totally right and was what my life was all about – caring for my beautiful daughter. I miss jumping out of bed in the morning, even though I had only had a few hours' sleep, because I was going to spend another day with my amazing little girl. Jumping in the shower and getting dressed as quickly as I could – I never once dried my hair with a hairdryer during Erin's life because that would just be wasting time. I could not wait to be by her side and every minute was precious. I miss getting up in the morning and saying excitedly to my husband, 'Come on, let's go and see our little poppet.' I miss changing her as she wriggled around on the mat – trying to work around the wires and monitors. I miss choosing a babygrow for her to wear and dressing her proudly. I miss everything!

The rest of Erin's life was spent in the ICU following an operation on her heart. This was a very different time as she was critically ill and there were no cuddles, or dressing or stretching anymore . . . but despite this, there was still hope. I still remember a skip in my step as I rushed down to the ward each morning, hoping that this would be the day when she would start to improve. There were still tremendous feelings of pride as I sat by her side, whispering words of comfort in her ear, stroking her hair and holding her hand. These feelings of pride will never leave me.

Then there are the things I miss that I never even got to do. I miss having the opportunity to sit in the rocking chair in her nursery with her and sing her to sleep. I miss having the chance to take her for walks in the sunshine and visit Daddy during his lunch break at work. I miss the fact that I never got the chance to introduce her to most of my friends and family and that she never got to enjoy all the cuddles she would have had. I miss getting out of bed full of hope and joy in the morning . . .

When we returned home from hospital without Erin, one of the first things I did was write down all the wonderful things about her – the details of her hair and her weight and the funny little mannerisms she had. I was so terrified that one day I might forget them and I never wanted to forget anything about my precious little girl. Now I know that I will never forget those things, but I do worry that I will forget how those things felt. I struggle to remember just how it felt to hold my baby girl close and this scares me, because my memories are everything; they are all I have.

It is seven years now since Erin died and I'm a different me. I live with more fear and I've accepted that I will grieve for her for the rest of my life. Even on the most joyous occasions, when I laugh and smile, I am mindful that she is not here. I feel sadness for all she is missing out on and I miss her desperately. I'll always wonder what our lives would have been like had she lived, and I'll always feel our lives are infinitely poorer because she didn't.

I will miss you until the end of time, when the sun stops rising and the earth no longer spins . . . even then my heart will crave to hold you.

ZOË CLARK-COATES

Loss of a Mother

It was only after my mum died in 2007 that I finally used the word that had stuck in my throat all those years and made me feel like I was always somehow living a lie – the word was 'alcoholic'. We skirted around this word for years, talking about how difficult she was, how unpredictable, but never really saying what she suffered from and what that made us all too – children of an alcoholic and all that this inevitably entailed.

I lived all my life up until that point waiting for the phone call to tell me she had died. There were so many times prior to this when I thought it would happen and it is a dreadful thing to have hanging over you, that one day the alcohol would win, and we would lose her.

Under the addiction there was a bright, witty, interesting and unique person. There was also a mother who has given me so many of the traits, interests and strengths that make me who I am today. I owe such a lot to her and will always be grateful for the rich, varied and generous way she chose to live and see the world.

Being brought up by her opened me up to such a wide variety of experiences. We held poetry evenings at our house, were always on demonstrations, protest marches and involved with politics, and my views were always respected and sought. She gave me the ability to think outside the box, to work for a better society for all and to trust that I had the resources in me I would need to accomplish something good.

With all of this, however, came the heartbreaking and daily struggles with alcohol. I grew up knowing never to approach her after a certain time in the evening, that the predictability, such as it was, ended around 7pm most evenings and then she would retreat into a world of drinking and isolation, a world you didn't want to disturb.

There were also the more extreme times when she would be found unconscious or passed out, and it would be up to me to help her come through. One such event occurred on my birthday, and led to me cancelling a party I had arranged for myself in order to yet again be my mother's carer.

So much of these years revolved around simply surviving for her, and it was only once I had moved out that I finally started to breathe and become myself for the first time.

Our relationship did, however, improve over the last few years of her life, for many reasons, not least of which was that I was no longer prepared to simply put up with the status quo of what we had become. A new mum myself, my priorities shifted, and I found that I no longer could be my mother's carer in the way I once had been. It was both liberating and terrifying to lose this identity, but ultimately it led to an honesty between us that we had not before experienced.

On the day I received the phone call to say she had fallen and slipped into a coma I braced myself for what had been coming all these years. Braced myself to say goodbye to this complicated, challenging, frustrating and yet much-loved woman, my mother.

In the end it took a week for her to let go before the hospital finally turned off the life support, and my brothers and I stood by her as she let out her last breath. It was peaceful and there was no pain involved, which I am forever grateful for, but even more than that there were for me no regrets.

I had long ago accepted who she was and the problems that engulfed her, and had found a way to integrate that into the relationship we found ourselves sharing at the end. It was never easy and very often painful, but what we had was finally real and finally actually okay.

In the months that followed I began to name the illness, and, as I did, to separate her from the alcohol. she wasn't just an alcoholic, she was a truly interesting and special person who had sadly fought all her life with low self-esteem, which she masked with alcohol.

Now, as I think of her, I can feel sadness and that I do genuinely miss her. We both worked hard to reach this point, but this battle was one that between us we won and that the alcoholism couldn't destroy. She remains my mum and she is missed.

Grief is a battleground, a war for the heart.

ZOË CLARK-COATES

Loss of a Brother

Just over 25 years ago, my life changed forever. I lost my brother in a tragic accident – only to me, it doesn't feel like 25 years; for me it often feels like it was yesterday.

My brother, Nicholas, was the life and soul, with lots of friends and a promising future ahead of him. That day, he was on his way home after a night out and, for a laugh, he decided to stick his head out of the car as it was moving. Unfortunately for us, his family and friends, that decision proved fatal. His head struck a signpost and our lives would never be the same again.

My big brother, who I worshipped, was only 18 years old. He was expecting his A-level results a week later and he had his whole life ahead of him. At 16, you don't think about losing a close family member and certainly not the person who you thought would be one of your best friends and your partner in crime forever. It is an unthinkable event that doesn't happen to you. That kind of thing happens to someone else.

It didn't quite sink in. In fact, I don't think it ever really has and I have always struggled to come to terms with the loss of my big brother. Not accepting this loss has probably been one of my downfalls with dealing with my grief.

I have accepted that we are not meant to know the meaning of life, we are not meant to know why these things happen, and it is futile to look for the answers as you won't really find them. What I *do* know is that I will *always* miss my brother and always think about him. People say time is a healer, but I will never be able to replace the void that he has left in my heart and in my life.

Following his death, seeing his life cut short so cruelly, I think it is fair to say I hit the self-destruct button. On the one hand, I was trying to numb myself to the pain and perhaps, on the other, trying to live my life to the full, for both of us! At that time, I was the life and soul of the party, just like my brother. Only those who really knew me, knew the pain that was lying behind my forced smile and joie-de-vivre persona. Unfortunately, when the party stops, the pain doesn't.

Luckily someone else saw through the mask and we fell in love. 'Why did he want me?' I asked myself. 'I'm not worthy of being loved like this.' But he broke down my barriers and reminded me I was. Grief makes you question your worth: why them, not me? You can only start to heal by lowering those walls and letting people back in.

They say it isn't the snake bite that kills you, but the venom that follows. The same can be true of loss and grief. If you ignore the bite/loss, pretend it didn't happen and don't address the venom/grief, it will slowly begin to poison you.

Meeting and marrying my amazing husband, having two wonderful daughters, has helped me to slowly fill that void. Nothing replaces that loss but slowly my heart was also filled with happy thoughts, creating new memories together as a family.

I often talk to my daughters about their brilliant, charming and funny uncle. Sometimes I watch them play and recall how I played the same games with my brother. It helps to keep him with me always.

As I write this, I am filled with so many emotions, some

painful, some heart-warming, but nevertheless memories of him I would never want to forget. For all the years I punished myself in my grief, I know now that my kind, loving and irreplaceable big brother would want me to try to let that pain go, celebrate his memory and be happy.

So, tomorrow, big brother, that is what I intend to try to do, for you.

When your bones, mind and soul ache,
you know you are grieving.

ZOË CLARK-COATES

Loss of a Baby Brother

One of my earliest memories is sitting on the hospital bed where my elder brother Thomas should have been, knowing that he was not coming back. I was eighteen months old. He had died aged four in another room, whilst waiting to be examined. His heart, weakened and weary from a lifetime of congenital heart disease, had ceased its beating. My feelings then were not of grief, for a small child does not know or comprehend grief; rather, they were of an overwhelming fear that now I was alone. It never once occurred to me that he has ceased to exist; I had no adult explanation of death, only an innocent instinct. This young certainty of his continued existence in some form has remained my reassurance to this day.

My brother died before I had even learned the difference between he and I. I still felt us to be one entity, rather than two individuals: brother, and sister. The clarity with which I remember his death, and him, at such a tender age – really no more than a baby – I consider to the greatest gift I could possibly have been given. I had of course, been 'too young to remember', and for years I doubted whether this memory was even real; perhaps I had simply imagined it to give myself something tangible in order to fit in with my family story.

So, the confusion, fear, and panic that accompanied his death haunted me for over twenty years until I was, by complete accident, given the space to grieve. It felt alien at first, talking about a grief that I had thought was only a figment of my childish imagination; but then, as I let it become more real, and I let my bruised and broken heart start to feel its sadness, I thought I would die from the pain, and the grief. The anger at him for abandoning me, the guilt I felt at being unable to save him from his pain, and too the guilt I felt at it being I who survived, and not him, all threatened to saw my already fragmented heart into pieces. But I screamed and wept and thrashed my way through it, until a gentle peace started to replace the agony.

I am still left with the sadness of course, that void of loss that nothing can fill, but the anger and the guilt have passed. The fear too is still there: the fear that I will surely be abandoned if I let my heart love again. Every time my boyfriend, who is in the army, is deployed on exercise, I am sick with the belief that he will not come back. It is almost a conviction, born from fear.

Not a day goes past that I do not long for my brother to walk over the horizon, to hold me in his arms and tell me that it was all a mistake. I know rationally that this will not happen of course, but I think that my heart will always hope.

Grief has a voice and we must allow it to speak.

ZOË CLARK-COATES

Alyson's story

Friday, 7 December 2018 will forever be the day that everything changed. I had spent the day dashing around doing everyday things. It was my children's Christmas fair after school and, as I stood waiting for my daughter to have her face painted, my phone started ringing and I had this strange feeling that something was wrong. As I took the call, I felt my whole world stand still. 'You need to get to hospital – Dad has collapsed.' I remember the seconds after, going into a panic, grabbing the kids who were trying to see Father Christmas; they didn't understand the urgency. I turned to a friend and asked her to have the kids so I could go.

I ran out of the school to my car and drove to the hospital, my heart racing, part of me thinking, I'll get there and he'll be sat on a trolley absolutely fine. I couldn't think about the alternative – not my dad, not today.

I pulled up to the hospital and ran to A&E. A receptionist took me through the waiting room. I looked up and saw I was standing outside the doors marked 'Resus'.

My heart was beating outside of my chest, I felt so sick. A nurse came and took me into a waiting room and I remember asking her, 'Is he awake?' Her reply and her face told me he wasn't. I asked her again, 'Is he awake?' and her words broke me: 'I'm so sorry but you need to prepare yourself for the worst.'

I screamed and broke into an uncontrollable sob. A lady who was in the waiting room too came and consoled me. I don't know who she was, but she held me until the doctors came. They spoke to me and explained that they did all they could, but they just couldn't save him. My heart broke into a million pieces. He was gone. I remember sitting in a quiet room on my own with him, holding his hand, waiting for my mum and brothers, sobbing . . . I couldn't believe it. I had seen him less than 24 hours before, I had been joking with him, I had kissed his stubbly cheek and said 'See you later'.

The days that followed were a blur. I just felt so numb. The shock of losing Dad had rocked my world. I spent hours searching for photos, videos and cards he had written, anything that would remotely remind me of him. Trying to work out what exactly happened to him.

As a family we pieced together that he had walked miles around a nature reserve, taking photos of the beautiful sun shining. In the following days we met one of the people who helped him. I sobbed when she told me she held his hand until the ambulance took him. I will be forever grateful for that.

Over the days and weeks, I began to journey this road of unexpected grief, trying to get through day by day, hour by hour. Trying to make sense of what had happened. At night I would lie in bed for hours not being able to sleep, reliving every minute of that day, reliving the day before. Thinking of all the things I should've said or wanted to say now.

As the weeks went by, I began to try to find my new normal in a world without my dad, which was something I had never envisaged. Each day is still so different.

I've learnt that my grief cannot be suppressed. If I need to cry, I cry. If I need to talk, I talk. If I need to laugh, I laugh. I just have to go with the way I feel and not put pressure on myself to have it all together. I know that we were so fortunate to have such an incredible dad. I miss him so much.

As the seasons change so does our grief, that's how nature shows us that the beauty of life is . . . that it goes on.

ZOË CLARK-COATES

Julie's story

Angela was more to me than my sister – she was my best friend for all of my life. There was a gap of only 14 months between us; Angela is in all my childhood memories. As children we always played together. We had other friends but were closest to each other. It is difficult to describe our bond but we got closer every year. Angela was there one way or another for all of the 43 years of my life until 26 November 2013.

Angela married her soulmate Ted and they had a beautiful daughter, Emma. Angela and Ted then went on to try for another child. Angela had five miscarriages; she found it devastating.

Angela went into hospital for a D&C [dilation and curettage] for the fifth miscarriage, and when she came round the doctor told her they could not carry out the procedure as Angela had a tumour on her cervix. Angela got Ted to phone me and let me know straight away.

I was off work on maternity leave, so was able to take Ange to appointments and help get Emma to and from school. It never occurred to me that Angela would not beat cancer. She was doing well and the tumour was getting smaller; however, Angela started getting blood clots as a side effect of the treatment. Angela did not respond to any of the blood thinners the doctors tried. It was like a ticking time bomb. Ted told me to spend every moment I could with Ange.

November 26th I was in work for 7am. I remember

sitting at my desk wanting to text Ange to see how her night had been, as she had had trouble sleeping, but I didn't want to send the text early in case it woke her. I eventually texted at 8am but Ange never read it.

I can remember every detail of that day, and in the end my counsellor advised me to write it down as I kept replaying it in my mind.

I don't know how I got through those early days of grief. I can remember throwing a glass across the kitchen out of frustration. My one-year-old daughter, who I first made laugh, picked up on my grief and always wanted Daddy.

I shut myself down; I don't know how my husband coped with me . . . I gave nothing back to him for at least 18 months.

I was off work for five months. Ange and I had worked together. Apparently, work is normally a good distraction, but mine was full of memories of Ange. I barely left the house. I felt safe there.

Running is my antidepressant. I used to run before I lost Ange and it was a great de-stressor, but now it's more than that. I often think about Ange when I am running and will have tears running down my face, but I need it to mentally cope with life without my sister in it.

It will be five years this November since we lost Ange. I do get more enjoyment out of life than I did, but the loss of Ange is always there. Losing someone before their time is hard; I have lost grandparents I was close to and I miss them, but it's not like Ange. I see a counsellor when I need to and think I always will when things get too much. It's the things Ange is not here for that hurt, even small changes, when I think, Ange won't see that. I see a lot of my niece Emma, she and Eva are like sisters, and

I would not have it any other way, but I am always conscious that Ange should be there on our days out too.

One of the things I find hardest is when people ask how you are. I always say, 'Okay', but want to say, 'Okay except for Ange not being here.' I find life without Ange in it very hard. My husband and daughter have saved me. Especially the joy my daughter has given me as she is growing up.

My life feels like it's been in two parts – before and after the loss of Ange.

〰〰〰〰〰〰〰〰〰〰〰〰〰〰〰〰〰〰〰〰〰〰〰〰〰〰〰〰

I used to feel lied to, as somewhere along the line someone led me to believe we were in control of this thing called life, now I know this couldn't be further from the truth. We are meant to fail, just as much as we are supposed to succeed. We are meant to rejoice over those being born, and we are supposed to weep over the ones that leave. We aren't meant to know the way, one of the most valuable parts of the journey is getting lost. This is life, this is the messy, beautiful, screwed-up world we reside in.

〰〰〰〰〰〰〰〰〰〰 ZOË CLARK-COATES 〰〰〰〰〰〰〰〰〰〰

Loss of a Friend

The loss of a great friend causes a deep ache that no one else can replace. Jane and I met right after I moved areas. I didn't have many friends in my new city and she had recently moved to the area as well. We became fast friends and it seems I can no longer remember a time when we didn't know each other. Me being a stay-at-home mum and her – her grown children already out of the house – working from home afforded us the opportunity to spend hours on the phone each day. We talked about everything from the stock market to dirty nappies She was one of the few people I trusted wholeheartedly never to judge me, never to make me feel badly, no matter what I told her. We laughed and cried so many times together. She adored my children and quickly became part of our family, sharing holidays, birthdays, anniversaries and just about any get-together or celebration with us. Jane was unbelievably energetic and full of life. She brought a light everywhere she went and there wasn't a soul alive who wasn't drawn to her. We spent our summers sitting on the beach and our winters visiting each other's homes just to sit and chat all day.

I remember like it was 10 minutes ago the day she was lost to us.

She called me at 9.30 that morning to tell me about something exciting that had happened. We talked for an hour or so and said goodbye. At 3.30 that afternoon, I called her to ask her if she'd like to join me and some friends at the movies that evening. She told me she was about to put dinner in the oven and take the dogs for a walk and that she was going to stay in that evening. We talked for about 45 minutes and once again said goodbye.

Two hours later I got a phone call from another friend of ours saying that Jane was in an ambulance and did I know her security code for her alarm system as the fire department smelled food cooking and needed to get into her house. I phoned her brother to let him know what was happening and to see if he had the code. He phoned me back an hour later and told me she was gone.

Gone. My mind went numb. How could someone I'd just had a conversation with simply be gone? Time started moving very slowly. I couldn't seem to wrap my head around the loss of someone so much a part of our everyday lives. Days passed, her funeral came and went, and still I had a hard time coming to terms with her absence. Jane was so full of life. Always lighting up a room with her contagious laughter and beautiful big smile. How could these things just be gone? With time the dust began to settle and still I struggled daily with wanting to pick up the phone and talk to my best friend. Summer came and went and it was a challenge to get through a season in which we'd enjoyed so much previously. My children asked where she was and with every question, I struggled with explaining death to a six-year-old and a two-year-old in a way they'd understand.

I tried desperately to hold onto the memories and time we had. In life we have only so many good and true friends. To lose someone so irreplaceable and integral to our life was a massive blow.

It's been almost three years since Jane passed and it hasn't gotten easier, only different. We walked through our grief and came out the other side forever changed.

Losing a best friend is a terrible feeling. Not having that person you can tell everything to, someone you can always relate to, the person who knows your deepest, darkest secrets and still loves you unconditionally. Someone you can always feel comfortable with and who you know will never judge you. These qualities which are so hard to find in people are held always by your best friend. We never truly appreciate the value of those moments until they are gone.

I still try to honour Jane each day, remembering and abiding by the advice she gave me over the years. I find time to sit and smile about the fun we had and cry over the trials we survived together. I will never find another friend like Jane and, truthfully, I don't want to. There are people who walk into our lives and leave such an imprint that not even death can make it fade. These are the people we carry forever in our hearts.

Grief asks you to leave your old self behind,
if you don't comply it mercilessly demands it.

ZOË CLARK-COATES

Don and Lynne's story

We lost our son, Dave, to suicide in November 2011.

He was the youngest of our four children – a good-looking, bright, funny, sensitive A-level student at sixth-form college and a great musician. We were a close family and thought that we were good at communicating. However, we were not aware of how desperate Dave was feeling – he was good at putting on an act and could be the life and soul of the party.

At 16, we knew he was feeling low having been bullied at school and having lost a girlfriend, and thought that talking to a doctor might help. He chose to go in on his own and it was only when we saw the details of this visit when preparing for his inquest that we realised he was feeling suicidal at that point. He didn't get any help at this time, but came through it.

At 17, Dave told us that he had made a doctor's appointment (five weeks before he died) and we were pleased that he was taking care of himself. We didn't delve into why he was going, but afterwards he simply said that it had been a waste of time. We didn't realise at that time that the doctor knew he was suicidal. There followed a whole series of human errors, system failures and communication breakdowns between the professional services and so he failed to get the help he needed.

On looking back, we felt that we were 'parenting in the dark' and, had we known, things could have been very different. Medical confidentiality is misguided when someone is at risk of dying – they need a network of help around them. We cannot stress enough just how important this is – leaving anyone isolated at a time when they need support the most is a recipe for disaster.

It is hard to describe the pain of losing a young person to suicide. The shock is tremendous and assaults your body and mind. The 'what if?' questions inevitably come – but there are no satisfactory answers. Nothing will bring Dave back. It would also be easy to apportion blame. But we realised that forgiveness is vital for our own well-being and for those responsible for errors.

In our case, there were resulting changes to operating procedures, and, hopefully, that will help to prevent others going through what we have. Also, it has prompted us to become involved with suicide prevention and we volunteer for the charity Papyrus, for the prevention of young suicide, as we are determined that Dave will not have died in vain. We tell our story whenever we can in order to help break the stigma around suicide in our nation. Suicide can happen in any family – it is the biggest cause of death in under 35-year-olds.

How did we get through? Our support for one another was important, as was keeping the whole family close so that we could mourn together. Our faith in God was, and remains, an essential source of hope for the future. We continue to talk about Dave a lot in a positive way and our children and grandchildren do too, even though the youngest wasn't even born when he died – he is still very much part of their lives. The pain never goes, but we try to create a 'new normal'. We continue to mark important dates in small ways, and we celebrated his 18th and 21st birthdays in his absence. If we are able, we would love to offer a little advice to others who may be walking a similar path, as if even one death can be prevented in honour of Dave, us sharing our story will be worth it.

- Look for changes in behaviour – are they spending more time by themselves, have they given up sports or something they used to be involved with?

- Is there a sadness, or are they more stressed? Maybe angrier or frustrated?

- Ask them how they are feeling, on a scale of 1–10. Have they felt suicidal? If they haven't, you can say that they can always talk to you if ever they do. It is important to get that word into the conversation. You will never plant a seed, but if it's there, it has made it okay to talk.

- Remain calm and try to get to the bottom of what is happening. Try not to react to whatever they say. Ask how you can help.

- Get help for them. Ring national helplines for advice.

- Go with them to the doctor and ensure that you don't get caught in the 'confidentiality trap'.

- Don't just assume it is mental health; we are holistic beings and everything contributes to how we feel. So, get a blood test to see if anything is wrong physically or if they are deficient in iron or other vitamins or minerals.

- If waiting lists are long, be prepared to get help privately, if you can. Be persistent. Go through this together but be sensitive to them needing space too.

- Usually many things contribute to a sense of hopelessness. Are there some pressures you can relieve them of? What do they love to do that will build them up? We all need to feel loved, accepted and secure. Assure them of your love and be patient with them. There is always hope – things will get better, but maybe they can't see that and need assurance. Stick with them for the long haul.

- Help them to practise being grateful and looking for positives each day. Look at nature, hear birds sing, look at the beauty around us . . . we need to feed our soul with good things.

I was meant to watch you grow old.

ZOË CLARK-COATES

Loss of a Friend

Mike's story

Picture the scene: two six-foot-three college lads and me, at five-eight, bombing around in my VW Polo Mk1, in a band (I was the drummer, Chris and Larry, lead and rhythm guitars); it was the late 1990s, cruising through the education system, getting ready to take on the world. Life didn't get much better.

Chris and Larry had grown up together; I'd only crashed the party when we started college, but we very rapidly became mates, really good mates, the kind of mates that turn into lifelong friends. By the end of the millennium we had finished our BTEC in media and the next phase was underway. I'd taken up a job in a local sound studio as a runner; Larry (that's not even his real name!) and Chris had both been accepted onto a degree course in sound production in Birmingham. The trio was separating but we would regularly meet up, either at their uni to record our latest track (wannabe rock stars with free kit and studio space), or back home where we would compare notes on our progression towards our dreams and ambitions. Eventually after three years they graduated – now the serious work could commence. While they had been in uni, I had started to climb the ladder at the studio, from lowly runner, to one of the recording engineers. We were all doing suitably well for ourselves, and if I haven't mentioned it before, life was good.

Then we had the news: Larry had landed a job at the BBC, by no means an easy thing to achieve for one so young. And Chris, this was the big one – he had been offered a job in one of the country's most renowned music studios. That just doesn't happen, people don't just get offered jobs in these places; they work, they graft, they go the extra mile to prove their worth and credibility. For these three lads from South Wales, life was exceedingly good.

It was Sunday night. Larry had settled into his job and moved to London, I was married, still at the studio moving up the rungs, and Chris was heading to bed, readying himself for his first day in the studio. Monday was going to be epic!

But Monday never came for Chris. He went to sleep and that was it. The report didn't find a reason. There was no logic or circumstances that would have caused him to die; he didn't smoke, wasn't a 'drinker' and drugs were never a thing. It should not have been him. But it was.

Almost 20 years on and I can still remember the phone call from Larry. Those words, 'Mate, Chris is dead . . .', the immediate feeling of emptiness. We spoke for a few minutes but I can't tell you what about exactly. My head was spinning. I sat down and tried to tell Claire (my wife) but my words barely formed. This had sucker-punched me. This wasn't meant to happen. Life all of a sudden had changed, and it was not good.

The funeral was rammed, standing room only. As hard as it was that day, it affirmed the fact that our mate Chris was a properly tidy gent. But that was the thing, he 'was', and now he 'wasn't'.

The next few days, weeks, months and years all manifested different feelings and responses. The aching question of why, the memories of the laughs and adventures we'd shared, the wonderings of what might have been his future – the job, a family, kids – it all seemed so unfair.

Blokes aren't supposed to get emotional, they're not meant to have deep-rooted friendships, and they sure as heck better not let those emotions out. But that is utter rubbish. Thankfully, I have my amazing wife, great friends and support. People who would just sit, sometimes in silence, sometimes to listen but many times to talk and laugh about anything and everything else. Larry and I still meet up, our paths cross professionally now; we still talk about the good old days. Chris is still a big part of that, he always will be. Sitting here and writing this hit me a lot harder than I thought it would. A lot of time has passed by but, when poked, those feelings are still there. Chris was a top bloke, a great mate and very sadly missed. My family has grown (we have four kids). Jobs have come and gone. Memories have been created and faded. But in all of life's twists and turns, the companionship of others, the willingness to stop and listen, the honesty to cry and not feel judged is the lifeblood of my humanity. And I truly am so very grateful for the life we have and the lives we connect with.

Grief makes you feel like you are unravelling.

ZOË CLARK-COATES

Gavin's story

Jill's death was as sudden as it was unexpected. She collapsed at home on the first working day of the new year. She died two days later in hospital having never regained consciousness. She had suffered a massive stroke – a subarachnoid haemorrhage.

A new year is a time for fresh starts. And 2017 was to have been a fresh start for both of us. We had lived at our home in Cannock, Staffordshire, longer than we had lived anywhere else. But for both of us it hadn't felt like home. Having spent the early years of our marriage moving about from one rented property to another, and from one part of the country to another, we made a promise that once our eldest son had started senior school we wouldn't move again until our youngest had finished it.

And so we ended 2016 and began the new year thinking about – but not quite planning – where we would move next: somewhere in the countryside, but not too cut off from amenities; somewhere close to the sea, but also within easy reach of London.

The fact that we hadn't actually planned anything didn't matter. We were enjoying dreaming dreams and imagining possibilities. Instead, those dreams turned to a living nightmare when Jill was taken from me.

That first night without Jill, I lay in bed thinking through questions which, at the time, I thought were pretty weird. I look back and they still seem weird: but I needed to know answers. Was I still allowed to wear my wedding ring? How long before I have to take it off? Who do I have to notify that my status is no longer 'married' but 'widower'?

That house we didn't like and wanted to leave was now a treasure trove of precious memories. When two people are downsizing, it is easy to throw away junk. But what if that junk is now an irreplaceable keepsake?

The year 2017 was supposed to be a new start in more ways than one. I was working on a freelance basis, and a major 16-month consultancy was due to finish at the end of January. We had been thinking about what I was going to do to replace it; and we had come up with some creative ideas. But now, my creativity had gone; as had my drive, my focus, my determination – and my will.

It wasn't only Jill that had died. A big part of who I was had died too.

I didn't want to go to bed at night because I couldn't sleep; but I didn't want to get out of bed in the morning because that meant I'd have to do things, anything, something.

The reality is that, while I never contemplated suicide, I desperately wanted to go to sleep and never wake up.

How can you plan for a future when you feel that you have no future? How can you take steps forward when you don't know what direction you are going in?

I don't know how I got from there to here; but more than two years on, I am in a much brighter and happier place. I know that I have a future, and I know what direction I'm going in; even though I do not know the final destination.

I have a good job and I'm engaged to a wonderful lady. I won't ever forget Jill.

I will hold in my heart forever the love that we had for each other.

I still grieve for her, and miss her desperately; but now I've given myself permission to carry on living again.

✎ ✎

It hurt when I was awake. It hurt when I was asleep.
Heck it hurt to simply breathe.

✎ ✎ ✎ ✎ ✎ ✎ ✎ ✎ ✎ ZOË CLARK-COATES ✎ ✎ ✎ ✎ ✎ ✎ ✎ ✎ ✎ ✎

Loss of a Child

Nicole's story

Our second son Ben was born happy and healthy at 39 weeks. He had the loudest scream – thank you, reflux – but the warmest smile, and he had me wrapped around his little finger. He was 100 per cent a daddy's boy and adored his big brother; every day he was told how much we all loved him. But on a cold Tuesday morning in November our lives were changed forever.

Having just moved to Scotland, I was on a mission to make mummy friends, so I took Ben and his older brother, Alistair, to the local toddler group. The morning was a huge success; the boys played, and I met other mums. At the end of the session I secured Alistair into the toddler seat on the top of the pram and slid Ben in his bassinet underneath. Ben was exhausted and fell straight to sleep.

As his eyes closed, I remember the look he gave me: pure love. I had no idea that would be the last time I would see his eyes; it is a moment I will treasure for the rest of my days.

After loading the pram up with shopping and visiting the local charity shops, I secured the rain cover over Ben's part of the pram and we walked home. When I got to my friend's front door, I went to get Ben out of the pram, but that is the second everything changed, our lives would never be the same. In the brief 10-minute walk home, the chicken for tea had slipped off the hood of the pram and landed on his face. Ben was not breathing; he was blue and floppy.

The smallest decision destroyed our world.

After giving Ben CPR, and my friend going and getting help, we were able to make him pink again but unfortunately the damage was done. Later that afternoon my husband and I were informed that Ben was not responding to treatment. We had to make the decision that no parent ever wants to have to make. We had to turn off our own son's life support. At 4.30pm on 13 November 2012 Ben took his last breaths surrounded by the pure love of his mummy and daddy. It was the most peaceful moment I have ever experienced and one that changed our world forever.

When Ben died we lost a future with him in it. We lost all the hopes and dreams we had, not only for him, but for our own lives as well. We lost who we were as parents, as a couple, as individuals. We lost our innocence. The safety of life is taken away once your child dies.

Child loss, in any form, is a taboo. It is against the nat-ural order of life, so we try to make sure that we are safe, and we try to make sure it never happens to us. All any parents want is to be able to take their baby home, because getting them home means they are safe. But what happens when you are the parent whose child has come home safely, was healthy and had a long future ahead of them, but dies in a freak accident?

You become the ultimate taboo! Why? Because if people acknowledge your existence, they will never feel safe again. Child death is the elephant in the room of any culture, but accidental child death is the elephant in the room wearing a tutu and shooting sparkles out of his trunk.

So how do you live, being the sparkle-shooting, tutu-wearing elephant?

We started at the very foundation of our lives, our marriage. My husband and I made a pact – that we would not give up on each other. The hardest thing that we have had to do is trust that we never mean to hurt each other. Living with grief is like living with an open wound; some days the scab is hard and it doesn't hurt, but other days your wound is open and raw. You must be gentle with yourself but also trust that others don't mean to make the wound worse. We take each day at a time and we tell each other, and those around us, when we are struggling.

Our families have learnt that we love talking about Ben; saying his name helps our grief. Talking about Ben helps heal our hearts. We will never be the same again, I have changed to my very core, but I am still a mum, I still love my child and I will always want to talk about him just as I want to talk about our other children. When I tell people about my son, I see fear in their eyes and that makes me sad. It breaks my heart a little bit more every time that people can't see past his accident. Ben was a beautiful boy who is loved and deeply missed. I don't want him to be remembered for how he died; I want him to be remembered for how he lived, all 122 days.

Your heart taught my heart to beat. Your eyes taught my eyes to see. Your ears taught my ears to truly hear. Everything about you, changed every part of me.

ZOË CLARK-COATES

Loss of a Mother

George's story

I am a 47-year-old married man. I consider myself to be very blessed. I have an adopted son who is nearly five years old. While parenting him is very hard work, due to circumstances out of all our hands, he brings immense joy and happiness every single day. I have a stepdaughter who I love dearly and, while I know I am not her 'dad', if anyone asks me about children I always reply that I have two. I am approaching ten years married now to the most beautiful person I have ever met.

I am self-employed and have been very busy for the last few years. Not long ago I volunteered to help on the BBC show *DIY SOS: The Big Build*, where I spent three days helping to decorate a new home. The family story struck a chord with me. Two children had lost their mother to cancer and were forced to live with Granny and their young uncle in a two-bed semi. Wow! Three days of hard work but the most rewarding and proud time in my working life. A weight had been lifted without me knowing it.

I don't know how I got here but I have. The old saying of 'life goes on' is true but it doesn't mean that things are easy – far from it. I spent the majority of my twenties and thirties in no-man's land. I pretty much floated through life and now think I didn't really stick at a job or relationship so as not to become too attached or relied upon. The feelings of self-doubt and not really wanting a connection ruled my life. I couldn't afford to lose that person again.

I was 10 years old, third of four brothers, and lost my mum to cancer. Life changed forever. While I was from a large extended Greek family where get-togethers were noisy and hectic, life was one of solitude for all of us boys. Too many mistakes were made. I don't blame anyone but that doesn't and didn't help. I kept asking why? I was quiet, confused, sad, angry and lonely, and felt cold, so cold.

My dad owned a takeaway so constantly worked – to be fair, it was his survival mechanism – so we only really saw him on a Sunday and by the end of the day too much alcohol took its toll. I talked to him about it a few years back and he asked what he was meant to do, he had lost his wife!

We were woken by an aunt that fateful morning and taken out for the day. Another aunt broke the news. By the time we saw Dad that afternoon we almost felt ashamed for crying when we saw him. Be strong, we were told – so we had to be. The funeral was the cruellest day of my life. The church was packed, wailing aplenty. My eldest brother was in a separate car with my dad. We three younger ones were in another car and, as we approached the cemetery, we pulled over to watch everyone go in. Apparently, we were too young to deal with it. Why couldn't we grieve? No goodbye when Mum passed and no goodbye when she was buried. The emptiness took over for a while, some years, but who's counting?

Some tough years followed and I didn't really focus on myself that much. If everyone around me was happy that would do for me. I put my feelings in a room and shut the door. I open it now and again and it can be very therapeutic when I do.

So where does this leave me? Years of sadness and pain, anger and upset. I look at myself today and I am content, but I miss her so much and just hope she would be proud of who I am today.

I would say to anyone: allow yourself to grieve, trying to keep the pain within helps no one; at some point it just has to spill out.

You don't know how deeply you will be affected by someone dying until their spirit leaves . . . in those first few agonising moments of silence you realise how intertwined your hearts were.

ZOË CLARK-COATES

Loss of a Grandfather

Fifteen years on from my papa's passing I visited the football club where he held a season ticket for 50 years. With memories of where he sat, I climbed the barriers hoping that old leather seat bearing his name would still be there.

As part of a conservation project the names of former season ticket holders were preserved, covered only by stickers. Everything stopped the second my husband said, 'Lindsay, I found it.'

I can't tell you how it felt to be able to sit with my arm around the chair he once occupied. I'm crying now just writing these words. With closed eyes, I breathed in the cold, Scottish air and could hear football chants. I could see him there, in his Gabicci anorak, Motherwell FC tie and flat cap. I could hear his raspy breathing from all the years of pneumonia. I could smell his aftershave and, most poignantly, I could feel his touch.

In a moment I was five years old again and he was teaching me to swim. With parents who divorced when I was a baby, my week was spent with my mum and my weekends with my grandparents where my dad would visit.

Everything I know how to do I learnt from him. Riding my bike, reciting poems, bartering for bargains, making his favourite sweet, Scottish tablet . . . Every Friday I would run home from school counting the minutes till my papa came to collect me.

I have a strange affinity with garden sheds because of

him. Just the smell of sawdust and creosote and I'm in a warm haze of childhood memories; safety, for me is associated with my papa.

I will never forget the day the call came. I was lying in bed having suffered a miscarriage, just six months after my wedding. He had plodded through my big day, even MCing the reception and doing a reading in the church, but a nasty bout of pneumonia was taking its toll. I had spoken to him and my gran just the day before, but as 'DAD' flashed up on my phone screen I knew instantly what lay ahead.

'What's wrong?'

'It's Papa . . . you need to come home.'

I wasn't well myself but jumped in my car. I took every wrong turn, on a road I knew like the back of my hand, such was the panic and the intensity of how I was feeling. I arrived at the hospital to a full room. The last to arrive, I sat by his side. 'I love you, Papa', 'I love you too . . .' And they would be his final words. As my gran cried, 'Don't leave me, George!' I felt my world collapse around me.

This man was my everything. I'm 17 years on from that day and it's as raw as it was then. When I look at my children, I imagine him with them. When I accomplish anything, I still pick up the phone to tell him. I regularly cry just remembering him saying, 'I fairly miss you, dear' when I left for college, and I'm still full of regret that there're no photos of him and me on my wedding day.

I haven't lost my parents so I can't compare, but I pray it won't be worse. My grief for my papa is mainly hidden now, but like a quiet shadow it's always there and some days it's so visible it's enormous. I've never forgotten him or the pain of the loss. If I'm honest, I don't want to.

> No one warned me about the huge grief surges
> that come from nowhere . . . they make you question
> your ability to survive the pain.

ZOË CLARK-COATES

Loss of a Wife

Raymond's story

I guess if you are married to your soulmate you dread the moment when life separates you, and the older you get the closer that day feels.

My wife had suffered with ill health her whole life, and so our marriage was filled with many moments where we thought a goodbye was inevitable. But due to amazing care by the NHS she always bounced back and that meant I got to hold her until she was 86 years of age.

Over 65 years of loving her, taking care of her, cherishing her, and in one moment she was gone. I barely left her side following her cancer diagnosis, but she died when I nipped to the loo. I guess it was too hard for her to slip away while I was beside her, and as always she knew best! Watching her fade away was heart-shattering, and I felt it almost impossible to be selfless enough to give her permission to leave, as I wanted her to stay forever.

Nothing could have prepared me for the weeks and

months that followed. Life lost its meaning, and even though I was surrounded by family that loved me, and whom I adored, the pain was so overwhelming I longed to just be with her in heaven.

They say silence is deafening and that is painfully true. When you suddenly live alone, the feelings of isolation become suffocating. You become aware of every little noise in the house, the hum of the freezer and the sound of every car driving by. That inane chat that is just part of life is gone, the simple 'good morning' and the quickly muttered 'good night' are painfully absent.

It took me at least two years for the shock of her passing to fade, and the pain of her not being here is as big today as it was then. I will never be used to her not being here with me, for I am part of her and she is part of me, but I have now got used to a new normal. Life now has a new meaning, and I have chosen to keep on living in her honour. I know she would want me to make sure all the family are okay, and I hope she is looking down on me and feeling proud of me doing just that.

In every second of every day I will search for you
until we once again share the same space.

ZOË CLARK-COATES

Loss of a Mother

Carys's story

Today marks two months since my mum suddenly passed away. It all started back in August 2018. I woke up one Saturday morning and realised I had overslept. I was supposed to be meeting my mum – we had planned to go look at a wedding invitation shop together, check out the new Sketchers shop, and then TGI Fridays for lunch. As I was dashing to the shower my phone started ringing and it was my dad. He could barely get his words out. Mum had suffered seizures during the night and had been rushed to hospital. We found out that her cancer was back, but this time it was tumours in her brain. She was told she had weeks to months left to live.

My mum didn't want anyone to know she was ill, never mind dying. We had to respect her wishes. It was so hard to keep quiet a situation that was going to change my life. I couldn't think of a life without my mum. I would cry more than once a day. I can remember telling my fiancé that I wanted to go with my mum when she died, because I didn't know how I would be able to function without her. I valued her opinion so much that I wouldn't even buy clothes in a shop without sending her a photo from the changing rooms.

The next few weeks and months were surreal because Mum seemed to be getting stronger. It was always in the back of my mind that she will never get better. I would always leave her thinking this could be the last time I see her.

My best friend passed away suddenly five months later after suffering another seizure when she was home alone.

I miss being able to text, call or FaceTime her like I did every day. It's the hardest thing ever to plan a wedding when her opinion is one of those I cared about the most. I want to be able to tell her about my day. She would also give me great support or tell me to get on with it on the days when I needed to be told that as well.

Being only 24, there have been some great moments in my life that I'm thankful my mum has been a part of, like my graduation, engagement, helping me move out even if it was just round the corner to the next street. Our houses are 0.1 miles apart. She was able to see me settle into a great relationship with my fiancé; she helped me pick out my perfect wedding dress and attended wedding fairs with me.

It brings me great sadness to think of all the things she will miss – my sister's graduation this summer, the actual wedding, being a grandmother in the future and seeing the next chapter of my life and my sister's life unfold.

I have started keeping a diary. It's just a plain 2019 one-day-a-page A5 diary. I write every day about all the things I would have wanted to tell her. Someone told me that the pain of not being able to tell my mum things will subside, and eventually it will be replaced with the happiness of thinking, 'My mum would have loved that.'

When we grieve we enter a world of vulnerability, don't be afraid to walk down the path, my friend.

ZOË CLARK-COATES

Rachel's story

Not long after turning 21 my younger sister came down with a cold and sore throat – little did we know that after collapsing and an 18-hour battle in intensive care she would leave this earth. Young, fit, healthy and vibrant. I remember the hospital like it was yesterday; I remember the first time in the resuscitation ward then drawing back the curtains and seeing her lying with taped-shut eyes. I remember the multiple machines and all of their beeps, the involuntary movements that they made her make, and I remember never knowing if it was good news or bad news that the doctors were telling us. It was at about 3.20am on my birthday that she passed away.

I remember thinking why? and how? and what just happened? The days, weeks and months that followed all blur into each other.

For the first few days we were surrounded by friends and neighbours; we had people drop off food and so much love was showered upon us. I don't remember crying lots, although I remember the distinct feeling of wanting to be able to cry, and somehow not being able to – I guess the overwhelming shock stopped me being able to. It wasn't long after her death that various feelings of guilt started to haunt me. Guilt that I hadn't stayed in the night before she died to spend time with her, guilt for going to work on the day she was taken into hospital, guilt that I wasn't crying as much as other people. Even after all this time guilt still creeps up on me. I will always wonder if I grieved 'properly' (whatever that means). I worry that I was too busy afterwards to grieve fully, and I worry that I still haven't processed it 'correctly' – and I question whether, if I haven't processed it correctly, that will mean that at some point I will have some sort of breakdown and have to relive it all again.

I chose straight after the funeral to get back to work and carry on as 'normal'. I booked in a wisdom tooth operation, went to lots of social things and busied myself any way I knew how. I'm not sure now if I would change that; I can see how it contributed to my recovery and to the choices I've made in how I talk about Lizzie and honour her. I can equally see how it fast-tracked me back into some kind of a normal life and I am not sure whether or not that was the healthy thing to do. I guess I will never know. You do what you feel is right at the time and that might look very different to what is right for someone else.

Everyone grieves differently and everyone has a different perception of grief. Watching your family grieve is the hardest thing; I found it harder than handling my own grief, to be honest.

Having people grieve on me over their loss was the strangest thing, and having people explain to me the severity of a parent losing a child often felt insensitive. I was watching that up close and personal with my parents and was painfully aware of it, yet, at the same time, it almost went to discredit my own grief. My parents must have felt the tension. Not long after, I remember them wanting a photo canvas of myself and my brother. With so many things given to them in remembrance of Lizzie, Mum said, 'I have three children.' She wanted some things of us in the house too.

Eight years on, the big grief blips are less frequent, but what is really difficult is how much life has moved on and changed, but yet there is a Lizzie-shaped hole in everything.

A few years ago, I had a horrendous night – I woke up feeling like I couldn't remember Lizzie anymore. In a wild panic I looked at photos of her and I felt like I couldn't pinpoint memories of our lives together, and that really scared me. That evening was probably only the second or third time in the journey of my grief where I felt like I was back at the very beginning of the grieving cycle. I wasn't, of course, but that is the nature of grief – it can catch you when you least expect it. I will always miss my sister; part of me went with her that day, but I now live to make a difference in her honour.

* *

Be patient with yourself as you grieve,
you are unfolding my friend.

ZOË CLARK-COATES

Loss of a Friend

Losing Hannah was a surreal experience. We'd been friends on and off since we were 17, bonding over a love of obscure French words and French culture in general.

When I got the call, time slowed down and the disbelief ramped up. Thirty-three-year-olds don't just fall down the stairs and die. The guilt kicked in: she lived alone; if I'd been able to visit right then would I have found her? If she'd told someone she had the flu maybe they'd have been with her instead of finding her days later.

I'd just been released from hospital the day before she died. Only we don't know the exact date of her death; instead, we have a three-day window from her last phone call to the day her body was found. In a cruel twist of fate, she was found on my wedding anniversary and now a happy date is tied inextricably with grief and sadness and loss.

I spent the first week in tears and shock; we had to wait for the funeral, which left me in a sort of paused state. I couldn't believe she was gone so kept searching social media for updates from her family. I had ironically to travel to France for a wedding while we waited to bury her, and it seemed crueller as I couldn't text her to share my news of surviving my first French wedding experience.

For many days after her loss I googled for news reports of her, seeking tiny details to add to the small fragments I knew. Reading her name in print brought comfort. I wrote messages to her on Facebook and emails which bounced back telling her I loved her and missed her.

The longer we waited for the funeral, the harder un-pausing became; then after the funeral came the wait for the inquest. Seven long months after she died, we finally heard what we already knew. It had been a terrible, sense-less accident.

The first day after the inquest I didn't know what to do; the wait was finally over but it didn't seem real yet. It wasn't until the first anniversary of her death that I really felt like she was truly gone. I realised I was the only one writing on her Facebook page commemorating birthdays and memorials, so instead switched to messaging her mother to make sure she knew her daughter wasn't gone from my mind.

Losing a friend in my thirties feels so wrong. We're almost five years down the line and writing this is still harrowing when I recall those first few weeks. But now on New Year's Eve, a night which we'd shared many times over the years, I can raise a glass and a smile instead of watching the fireworks with tears in my eyes. I won't forget her, there's still a hole where she should be, but if I'd not continued forward, learning more obscure French words and trying to teach them to my children, I'd be losing her twice over.

When it hurts this deeply, you know it matters that much.

ZOË CLARK-COATES

Loss of a Friend

Last summer I lost a childhood friend, albeit in the body of a 32-year-old man. There's something wrong with people in their thirties dying, especially strong, fit healthy ones who die in random accidents.

I found myself in a state of disbelief, anger – it couldn't possibly be true! He was so young, so fit, so well. No there must have been a mistake!

This internal battle with myself went on for two weeks. The funeral had taken place abroad so we waited for the memorial service, which made me rage as well. I was scared I'd not be able to move on without a body in a casket and in the first two weeks no tear had been shed.

I didn't sleep, food was bland; I walked many miles on an evening trying frantically to exhaust myself so the sleep would come, but still it eluded me. I talked to his siblings, other childhood friends of mine; they shared my disbelief and we formed an alliance of disbelievers. We recounted tale upon tale of hilarious mishap and brave endeavours, of postcards sent home with clever riddles that took an age for us to work out.

But still the sleep didn't come easily. A beautiful memorial service passed and still the tears didn't come, still the miles were walked. And then one evening I got lost. I took a wrong turn and grew angry with myself, then grew angry with the world, and the more enraged I was, the faster I walked, until finally exhausted and spent I cried. Out loud on the side of the road. Angry, fast, heart-wrenching sobs. That night I finally slept.

I'd love to tell you I woke up the next morning and felt better but I didn't. I struggled to enjoy things and felt really wrong with the world until one day I realised I didn't. Many weeks after his loss I finally felt a small part lighter. I finally enjoyed the scenery of an evening walk.

Grief – when day and night merge into
one and time loses all meaning.

ZOË CLARK-COATES

Loss of Grandparents

Andy's story

I had never gone through loss as a child, and was fortunate to enter my teenage years with a full complement of grand-parents. One set lived in the same area and we saw them perhaps once a month, while the other set lived about 70 miles away, which was a full day's trip in the car, so we only saw them two or three times a year. I loved both sets of grandparents, maternal and paternal, but I suppose I took them being here for granted, and it was not until I was 15 that it changed.

I was at my Saturday job when my parents' car pulled

up outside and I was told my nan had just passed away. I was upset, but like most teenage boys, you get on with life, with school and friends being a good distraction.

When I was 18, I joined a theatre company and toured the UK for two years. During this time one grandad became ill, and I drove the 300 miles to the hospital. What greeted me was a frail, elderly man, who was now a fraction of the man I remembered. He passed away hours later.

A couple of months later my second grandfather passed away, while I was on tour. I hate to admit it, but this felt almost 'normal', as I had almost resigned myself now to my grandparents passing away. Everyone said, 'Well, they are a good age', 'It's better they are not in pain', and so I fell into that thinking.

At 21, I married, and my new family included three grandparents on my wife's side, who were considerably younger than my grandparents had been. Within months, my last nan, who was disabled and who had suffered with ill health for years, developed dementia and then passed. I will never forget the final time I saw her as she no longer knew who I was . . .

Four years passed before my wife's grandmother sadly died, and now being much more mature, I began to understand loss and grief for what it was – a deeply painful and life-changing event, but something from which you could learn.

It was almost 15 years before my wife's other nan passed away, and I had become closer to her than any of my biological grandparents – I loved her like she was my blood relative. In the years before she passed, my wife and I had experienced brokenness, pain and grief from multiple baby losses which had brought us to our knees. We had been through those darkest nights, wailed in desperation, and come through the other side, still ourselves, but irrevocably changed. Because of these losses, I knew that this time I needed to let grief take me on its journey. I allowed myself to embrace the heartache, and allowed the tears to flow, as we grieved for Nan.

A few weeks ago, our final living grandparent passed away. He had been in my life longer than any of my maternal or paternal grandparents, and he wasn't just a grandparent, he was an amazing friend, who taught me so much. It was such a gift to help care for him in his final weeks and days on earth, enabling him to stay at home where he wanted to be. As a family we truly walked with him to the heavenly gates, and even though we didn't want him to leave us, we knew he was ready to rejoin Nan.

Grieving all my grandparents has taken nearly 30 years, and each loss has been processed so differently. I would encourage everyone to be real about their pain, and not to listen to the cliché that men don't cry, as I truly believe real men do cry; they allow themselves to feel all emotion, and that's how you become a compassionate human being.

~ ~

At times we aren't meant to know why, sometimes
the loss holds those secrets in its hands . . . we then just
have to learn to find peace in the unknowing.

~ ~ ~ ~ ~ ~ ~ ~ ~ ZOË CLARK-COATES ~ ~ ~ ~ ~ ~ ~ ~ ~

Jennalise's story

I remember the day so clearly and if I close my eyes I can almost feel my body collapse like it did on the 11 November when I got the call abroad from my dad that my dear 20-year-old brother James had died. I was alone at the time and pleaded and sobbed with my dad that he was wrong and perhaps there was more they could do.

I had just moved to London from Seattle, as I was only weeks away from getting married to my English fiancé Toby. The depth of pain and grief to follow were unbearable. I carried so much guilt about leaving my brother to move to the other side of the world. The next day I had to fly back to the States to help with the funeral and navigate the tricky relationships with my divorced parents and step-parents. I had to deal with so many questions and uncertainties – would I see my brother in his coffin, would I speak at his funeral, who would get his ashes, how would I cope mingling with the 500-plus guests at his memorial, etc.?

My soon-to-be husband was my anchor in the season to follow. Our wedding was shortly after the funeral and our first year of marriage was very hard and so unfair. My brother was meant to walk me down the aisle, so there was a moment in our wedding when we lit a candle to remember him. I was then on antidepressants for six months and I never left our house – we ended up living with my in-laws as the grief was too much to cope with. This is not what you dream of, being a newlywed! It was also very hard to live in a country where people don't talk about death or grief.

I was desperate to talk to people about my brother but it always felt like they didn't know what to say and it was always awkward. After about a year of sadness, going to bereavement counselling and my English family bringing me back to life, I slowly began to see light again.

It's been 10 years now and a lot of things still make me tear up and I still miss him so much. It's still hard flying to the States to see family and he's not with us. Not only have I grieved for my only sibling but also for a possible sister-in-law, nieces and nephews, family gatherings and, in the future, the support we'd give each other when we lose our parents. Losing my brother changed me so much – I now love more deeply and care less about materialistic things. I can't wait to hug him again someday. Now when I have a friend lose someone they love, my heart just aches for them, as the familiar feeling of grief just never goes away no matter how long it's been, but you just learn to cope with it and hold onto the hope of heaven someday.

It was as though part of my heart was broken
off . . . severed, detached, shattered.

ZOË CLARK-COATES

Margaret's story

At 60 I thought I knew about grief and could handle it fairly well, keeping control of my emotions. Then I discovered a different sort of grief. As a child, I had lost my father and brother; then as an adult, my mother, stepfather and parents-in-law. But nothing prepared me for the grief of losing my youngest child. She was 21 at the time and really just at the beginning of life's journey. Her features were changing as she became a wonderful young adult, and then it was over.

Her sudden death impacted me like nothing else ever had. A friend described what I was going through at first as numbing confusion. The floods of tears were still to come but initially I felt numb. I couldn't function properly. I couldn't remember whether I had showered, changed, eaten. This is where my friends, Lizzie's friends and both our churches stepped in. One rang every morning to check on me and make sure I had eaten. Others cooked us meals in those first days and others chauffeured me around as they didn't think I should drive.

As I came through that stage the tears started, usually at inconvenient times – in the middle of a shop or a street, as well as the private meltdowns. I was a completely changed person. I surrounded myself with photos of Lizzie. I started to use her purse and cling onto her things. Except her bed! Where this irrationality came from, I don't know, but in my mind I blamed the bed for her death. It was a high sleeper and perhaps I was thinking that if she'd collapsed in bed, she would have died there. All I know is I had to get it out of the house. A friend came and dismantled it and put it in his loft.

As time passed, I returned to some kind of normality. However, there's a massive hole in my life and in our family where Lizzie was. The first Christmas without her was torture, similarly the first Mother's Day and all the special dates. Several months later, I was at a function and must have looked sad. Two well-meaning friends told me I should be over my grief. That was like a slap in the face! I went out to the car and sobbed. You can't put a time limit on grief. I can't stop missing and loving my daughter. I can rebuild a life without her as I have no choice. Please never tell someone they should be over their grief. For everyone the recovery process is different. I need my photos; other people hide photos for a while. We each have to do what is right for us. It's a horrible road to tread and we all have to find our own path. There's no right or wrong way.

People say to me I paint a bleak picture but that's not my intention. Honesty is best and it's no good me telling another grieving mum that they'll be fine soon. It takes time, life goes on and you start to enjoy things again (and feel guilty for that at first!). However, for me there's always that feeling that part of me is missing.

I know you are probably wondering if the shattered pieces of your heart will ever function again . . . I promise you they will. Your heart will just be a very different shape than it was before.

ZOË CLARK-COATES

Jody's story

I lost my dad in October 2011 and I miss him every day. In February of that same year, Dad was feeling unwell and, while at the doctor's, his lung collapsed. He was rushed to hospital and eventually diagnosed with terminal lung cancer and given six months to live. I think my grieving started then.

It was a long, busy, drawn-out, rollercoaster of a time, from diagnosis to his passing away. He was mostly functioning up until two weeks before he died but needed help with washing, preparing meals and just having someone there. I would be with him almost every day and would feel guilty when I wasn't. Juggling emotions, time and everyday life, including family and work, really starts to wear you down and you feel like you are drowning under it all.

The last two weeks were horrendous, but the final few days, unbearable. I remember sitting on the toilet in the bathroom, crying my eyes out, texting a friend and saying, 'I don't think I can do this.' She told me I could, prayed with me and, of course, I carried on. Watching your lovely dad go through that breaks you. I hated thinking and feeling it, but I wished the end would come so that he wasn't suffering anymore.

And then he died. My world shattered. I felt guilt, sadness, anger . . . and relief that, finally, he wasn't in pain or feeling humiliated, or that we would have to see him in that way anymore. And then came more guilt for feeling those things. I also felt bereft and without purpose. My purpose for the last six months had been my dad. How did I function now?

We had support from family and friends and I also have faith, so found comfort in that. But we suffered a lot more loss in the year to come – two babies and my father-in-law, so the grief stored up and I didn't deal with it all immediately. It was a long journey but I can now talk and think about my dad with fondness and happiness. One of the hardest things to battle in the time afterwards is replacing the memory of the last few days with good ones from happy times shared in the past. What helped for me was talking about the good times with family and people who knew him, as well as looking at photos to remember him as he was, and not in those final moments.

It doesn't happen overnight and every journey is different. You just have to be kind to yourself, take one step at a time, but you *can* do it.

It was effortless to love you and the hardest thing in the world to lose you.

ZOË CLARK-COATES

Grieving While a Loved One Is Still Here

A question I often get asked is this: Is it actually possible to grieve for someone while they are still here? And the simple answer is yes, of course it is possible. Remember, grieving is a process and it is made up of thousands (or potentially millions) of layers. This process can begin at any time, and it certainly does not need someone to have died for it to start.

For many people the first time they encounter grief is when a friendship or a relationship breaks down. They feel this huge weight of sadness as they try to come to terms with what they are losing, and this pain, these complex feelings we often find hard to explain, that is grief. Grief from losing something or someone when all you want to do is hold on. Grief from losing a special connection that you have carefully built.

If you know someone you love is dying or has a long-term illness with a poor prognosis, grieving commences. Likewise, if someone you love is changing, due to health or for other reasons, you can experience grief because that person is no longer who they once were.

So how do we deal with this type of grief? In exactly the same way as we process grief once someone has died: we talk about it, we face it head-on, and this allows our brain to come to terms with the situation and the pain we are experiencing.

Grief =
A million what ifs
A billion if onlys
A trillion I wishs

ZOË CLARK-COATES

3
Practical Considerations

FEAR AFTER LOSING SOMEONE YOU LOVE

One of the legacies of grief and loss that is so rarely discussed is the fear that can consume you once the initial shock of the death has passed. This is even more acute in those who have had to watch a loved one die in front of their eyes over a period of time, as their fight-or-flight response will have been raised. Your stress hormones, adrenaline and cortisol, are always pumping, and your brain is waiting for you to face the worst-case scenario. Even once the loved one has died it is super-hard to switch off this response, and it can take years to master controlling it, but sadly most people just learn to live with it rather than stopping it dominating their lives.

Once you have lost someone you love it is also common to become hyper-protective of the loved ones that remain. At times this overprotectiveness can make a person look paranoid, sensing disaster at every turn. For example, a person behaving 100 per cent rationally would see a seagull sitting next to someone as a sweet photo opportunity. A person who lives with constant fear might see that seagull as a vulture, with the potential to peck their loved one's eyes out and possibly carry them away! While I can laugh at myself for thinking irrationally, and even find humour in being able to twist an innocent moment into a potentially dangerous situation, I constantly fight this fear, and have to choose not to be too overprotective, but it's not easy. We all need to accept that our natural response is to want to wrap the people we love in cotton wool, but as we don't want anyone to carry false fear and our hope is that everyone can live their lives to the maximum, we have to remind ourselves to step back and not project our fear on others.

Post-loss fear is so terribly hard to live with, and choosing to trade in that fear and hold onto hope will really help you move forwards.

If you give in to it, it can slowly take hold of so many other areas of life, so it is essential to silence the mind and refuse to allow it to capitalise on every little worry. A few common fear areas which people often struggle with post-loss include:

Fear of illness for yourself or others

This can be overwhelming and all-consuming. It can be concerns over little things or big things, and every symptom is overanalysed. When a person's imagination gets involved, even a common cold can look like a life-threatening condition.

I can't even begin to tell you how horrible it is for those who suffer with this fear, as it truly robs life of all joy. I always recommend people to have counselling or cognitive behavioural therapy (CBT) if they are suffering with this fear, as the quicker this pattern of thinking is stopped, the better. Being crippled by the fear of illness can be as bad as actually having the illness they fear.

Fear of accidents

This is another fear where the imagination can take you to some very dark places. Someone tells you they are just popping to the shops and will be back in 30 minutes. However, in that time you have already imagined they have been involved in a head-on collision and you are sitting waiting for the police to knock on your door to break the bad news to you.

There are some key skills to stop this cycle of thinking and the main one is to nip the negative thought in the bud the moment it rears its head.

Don't allow yourself to even enter into the dialogue in your brain. So, the second you think 'what if?', choose to think of something completely different. Once you start down the path of the accident, you are engaged in the thought pattern, so divert the thought, think of anything but – for example, what shall we have for supper? What would Lisa like for Christmas? You need to do a 180-degree turn. Eventually the negative thoughts should stop surfacing. If they don't, consider having some counselling.

Fear of bad news

This is very similar to fearing accidents and the same applies. Nip negative thoughts in the bud and don't engage with this spiral of fear.

Fear of going out

Sadly, this is quite common post-loss. Home can quickly become a safe place, somewhere a person feels they can be real and authentic, while the world outside can seem scary and fast-paced. Although it's fine to take time out and to hide away in our homes, we need to be careful that we don't avoid going out for too long, as this fear can really sneak up on you from nowhere. I always recommend simply going for short walks or brief drives regularly, so you at least see outside of your front door, and this can help avoid agoraphobia creeping in the back door.

Fear of socialising

This may start because a person has been in a situation where someone has said something painful to them, or it may start because they fear that they can't be real or authentic to themselves or their pain in the presence of other people. Either way, it's another fear that's better to fight early on, as the last thing you want is to become a recluse if you have previously loved being with people and socialising.

I suggest you start gently and spend time with those most likely to be sensitive and kind, then slowly expand your social circle. Remember, it is okay to realise certain people were never really your friend, or a kind person. I call grief 'the great revealer' – it's like a massive sieve and it brings so many issues and realities to the surface, and a common thing post-loss is finding out that some people aren't as lovely as you thought they were. So be mindful of this, especially if that has prompted your fear of socialising to develop. If your fear does continue, counselling can really help.

I urge you not to remain walking in fear, however that terror manifests itself; there is help available. It is possible to fight all fear and deal with it, even if that inner voice is yelling at you that it's not possible. Walking through life carrying this burden is truly debilitating – it is like having chains wrapped around your ankles. It shackles you, and I want you to be free!

Sometimes people become so good
at hiding their pain the world assumes they are
no longer suffering at all.

ZOË CLARK-COATES

INTIMACY (OR LACK OF) POST-LOSS

As you will be able to appreciate, this is an extremely tricky subject to tackle, as not only does the type of loss you have encountered play a part in the resuming of intimacy, but personality and your relationship with your partner will also affect your response and feelings about re-engaging at an intimate level. What I can say is that nothing and no one should force you into any physical intimacy before you feel ready and willing.

Firstly, let me say that lack of interest in sex or intimacy is incredibly common post-loss. When your world has imploded, just getting dressed can feel a challenge, let alone anything more physical, so if your interest in sex vanishes overnight, please know this is normal, and nothing to worry about.

So where do we start?

Perhaps a good place to commence this conversation is to talk about hugging and holding hands. For some, they need this physical touch to feel loved and cared for; for others, they don't want any physical contact, as they feel safer being in a bubble. This is something that needs to be discussed between partners (also with families and friends who may want to hug you), to ensure everyone's needs and expectations are being met. Where it becomes difficult in all areas of intimacy (whether it be basic physical touch or sexual intimacy) is when one partner feels one way, and the other feels very differently. What can you do if one party feels a need to have sex to feel loved and cared for, but the other can't even cope with the thought of it? The only answer to this is to talk about it. Not in order for one party to convince the other to do what they want, but so all feelings can be expressed and heard, as it's important to understand what page each person is on. Over time, and with much discussion, there is a chance that both people may feel a similar way. If, however, it becomes an 'issue', and a marriage/relationship is in danger because of it, I would always suggest seeing a counsellor, as having a third party involved with the discussion can help bring greater understanding and clarity.

Sex post-loss can be truly difficult emotionally; with this in mind, expect tears and be willing to talk about and share your feelings.

I always encourage people who fear intimacy post-loss to start slowly – imagine you are going back to the dating stage of your relationship. It can sometimes even be good to take sex out of the equation, and say no sex at all for x amount of time. This can be really helpful to some, and knowing there is going to be nothing more on offer than a kiss and a cuddle can remove all pressure.

Of course, there will be others who want to have sex and intimacy as quickly as possible, and that too is totally understandable. I know people who have said the sex they had post-loss was the best they'd ever had, as there was an intimacy there that they had never experienced before. When you feel at one with your partner, it can bring a sense of the pain you are feeling being emotionally shared, and this can make you feel less alone in your suffering.

My top tips:

- Talk to a loved one
- Take medical advice if you are worried about your libido vanishing or changing
- Take it a step at a time and don't let anyone rush you
- Don't be afraid to show emotion (intimacy post-loss is *always* super-emotional)

Now there is another side of this we need to discuss and that is when a person has lost their partner, so this part of their life is instantly removed from them. One day a person may be in an active sexual relationship, and the next they are forced into a period of celibacy, and for others there is the knowledge that they will be celibate for the rest of their lives – how does anyone come to terms with this?

Many people say the lack of sexual intimacy doesn't even occur to them for some time post-loss, as their sole focus is on surviving without their life partner by their side. But after a period of time this loss of intimate touch can become another thing to mourn, and that is what should be done. You have full rights to grieve for this; it is something else you have lost and often a subject that is not discussed. Most people are created with a sexual appetite, and when your partner dies and you lose the ability to satisfy these totally natural feelings, it can be very hard to deal with, especially if you feel it is not something you can openly discuss with family and friends. If you are struggling in this area please consider having some counselling, so you can be real and honest about the feelings you are experiencing.

Here are some stories from people about their experiences with intimacy post-loss.

Nikki's story

My name is Nikki and I am 36. Three years ago, on 7 March, my then husband sadly passed away. The cause was cancer – he was 37.

We married in a beautiful beach wedding in Jamaica on 28 August. He was an amazing man. We were very close, shared everything, travelled the world together, and lived a very fulfilling, fun life together.

I was absolutely shocked when he passed as he was so young and seemed so strong until the very end. I could not fathom life without him. When he passed I was broken. I remember feeling our 'connection' break as he passed, and his face as he knew what was happening and could not do anything to change the inevitable.

I was then introduced to a heartbreaking loneliness as I drove from the hospital with my parents that day. Waking up the next day I realised that this nightmare was actually my new life . . . The hopelessness was incredibly real, cold and scary.

The love from my family was very powerful in restoring hope and gave me a reason to live. I love travelling and was invited to visit Toronto – this was a huge help (the change of scenery), which turned into a US road trip which was amazingly healing for me. Gradually, day by day, I was reminded of things I loved.

I now am full of hope, thriving in the things I love again, and for a long time I did not think that was possible.

A very real thing I missed when my late husband passed was sex. This didn't start until around two years afterwards, but as my heart began to heal, I did begin to not only think about it but miss it!

I plan to wait until I am married again before having sex. Yes, it has been very hard after becoming so used to having sex regularly (being married) to now adapt to this new sexless life, but I hope one day I will find someone special to marry.

A very real and practical thing I found which helps me is to replace movies and songs etc. which show or talk about sex with 'clean' alternatives, as this helps keep thoughts about sex out of my head.

Living without sex is hard, but, I assure you, it is possible to survive without it.

From my first date with Susi I have never struggled to express my love and affection, holding hands, even kissing in public. It has always been something I've enjoyed more than anything. Being with Susi made me feel complete, excited, and, to borrow clichés from the worst of romance novelists, those early days of our relationship were charged with an electric intimacy.

A year into our relationship, we experienced two losses in what was, looking back, an incredibly short space of time. Anyone who goes through a similar loss will probably tell you that at the time every day feels a very long time. With the sadness of loss, the intimacy that we shared changed, the exciting rush, the tingling intensity developed into something deeper. Where before it had been an exciting, sensation-charged intimacy, a deeper, more protective dimension developed.

Within the year, we were married, had moved to a new house and were blessed with the birth of our daughter. All within the space of a couple of months. Throughout this often-stressful time, the intimacy of our love was something that made our relationship stronger. I haven't really realised or acknowledged that the feeling of a need to protect Susi has been there ever since. I still get that rush of excitement, that feeling in my chest whenever we're together, but it's a lot deeper and more mature than it was for that same guy 17 years ago.

I have never struggled with being close with my husband. We are very 'touchy-feely', hugging, always holding hands, and have never had a problem with public displays of affection. And I have loved him deeply since the moment we met.

After grieving two losses in a short space of time, I found that the intimacy between us changed and it was like a rollercoaster for me.

I found that my emotions were all over the place; we were closer than ever, but, also, I found that I was closing myself down (self-preservation, in my eyes). My husband was kind, gentle and loving, and giving constant support emotionally. We would cuddle together at night, but I would feel that I wasn't ready to go any further than that for what felt like quite a while. I just wanted to be held. Intimacy changed, for me.

My husband was so loving and patient and would hold me close every minute he could, and he made me feel safe.

We will never forget those times of loss, but we have grown together through this and I believe it has made us stronger. Being gentle with each other, taking our time and showing love is what helped me through this time. I would advise anyone to just take time for each other, it really works.

I'm not a touchy-feely person. Physical touch has never been my love language, and when I was growing up I would squirm uncomfortably when the time came to dole out the required hugs at family gatherings. Of course, all that changed when I met my husband. He was tall and muscular, with perfectly smooth tanned skin and the thickest, softest dark hair. He never let me get away without a hug – he would pull me against that rock-hard chest scented with Giorgio Armani cologne, and I didn't mind one bit. That was one place I would stay forever.

We had some difficult personal losses before the catastrophic day that ripped him away from me forever. I remember the day that we put my cat of 13 years to sleep. I crawled into bed, sobbing and heartbroken, and he, wordlessly, wrapped himself around me and held me for hours. The day I heard at a routine ultrasound appointment that our first baby had died at 12 weeks, he told me to stay in the parking lot until he could get there. He climbed into the passenger seat of my car and we held each other and cried. He was figuratively and literally my anchor in the storms of life, my soft place to land, the warm body cradling me at night, the hug or kiss or hand squeeze just when I needed it most.

My labour to bring our daughter into this world was 18 hours of unmedicated misery. The one thing that kept me from begging for an epidural was the conviction that my husband and I were in this together. He physically held me up through every contraction. He was the steady voice in my head with the unflagging reminder to 'relax' and 'breathe'. He held my hand while I slept fitfully, supported my aching back, held my legs while I pushed our daughter into the daylight. He was so physically *there* and a part of the experience that I knew I never could have done it without him.

When my soulmate died, the better part of my self died too. The tenderness and intimacy that he had awakened in me lay crushed on the highway with him. He had been my first kiss, my first lover, my first everything. Now it appears he will be my *only* kiss, my *only* love, and I will spend the rest of my life alone. But rather than terrifying me, this bleak prospect is oddly comforting. What we shared was such complete unity and so otherworldly that I cannot begin to fathom recreating it with anyone else.

I've been a widow for nearly five years now, even longer than I was a wife. I have surrendered to the dark valley of loss and come out on the other side. I've nurtured the fragile vein of vulnerability in my relationships, allowing myself to know and be known and receiving comfort in turn from my highly affectionate daughter – who inherited the love language of physical touch from her daddy! – and a multitude of family and friends. I have learnt, in spite of the grief that paralysed me for so long, that there is life beyond loss – life beyond sex. My marriage and my widowhood do not define me. There is a sun shining on me and a pulse of great purpose still beating deep in my heart, as dreams for the future propel me forward into possibility.

Due to my wife's poor health sex hadn't been possible for many years, so we lived a celibate life for quite some time before she died. However, when she passed away I grieved not being touched by her. You take for granted having someone to hug, a hand to hold, someone to stroke your back when you are feeling poorly, and when that goes overnight it's a huge shock. I guess we are created to crave human connection, and from childhood we are used to being held when we are weeping. Not to have that person you so desperately want to hold you, when you are the most broken you have ever been, is monumental.

It's been years since my wife's passing, but I still miss her embrace. I miss her not reaching out from her side of the bed to check I am there. I miss her rubbing my back and running her hand through my hair. I know this personal, intimate touch is not something I will ever experience again, and that adds extra weight to my grief, as I haven't just lost the love of my life, I have also lost so much more.

Loss changed me so dramatically that I thought physical intimacy was a thing of the past. I didn't know who I was any more, so how could I allow my partner to get that physically close? I couldn't have been more wrong though, as this new me, over time did enjoy sex again. In fact this new me enjoyed sex more! Loss made me feel things more deeply, and that included a new greater enjoyment of sex. I feel the boundaries that I once felt bound by were broken, a new found freedom was gifted to me, and no one could be more surprised about this than me. My message to anyone reading this would be if you feel scared, let me encourage you to take time to recover emotionally, and your body may surprise you down the line, like mine did with me.

RETURNING TO WORK

Returning to work after loss can be petrifying. It's a daunting thing to do after the loss of any loved one. Loss changes you, yet when people return to work they are often expected to be their old selves, which can be challenging.

Some people are entitled to paid bereavement leave, whereas others aren't even entitled to a single day of paid leave, and this is another huge challenge. People need time to recover both physically and emotionally, and only you know how much time you feel you need or want to take off work. If you aren't automatically given bereavement leave but you need time off, please book an appointment with your doctor. While they can't force your employer to pay you for time off, they can give you a doctor's sick note. Sometimes doctors write down depression as the reason for needing time off, and I often hear from people who resent this, as they so rightly tell me, 'But, Zoë, I am not depressed, I am grieving and there is a big difference.' Sadly, however, many doctors won't or can't list grief as a reason for time off work, so depression is often cited instead. The important thing here is that you have the space to recover emotionally, so if you are able financially to take time off, do consider it.

A note for the self-employed: I know this advice will come down to finances, and whether your work and clients will wait for you to return to work – sometimes jobs don't allow for any leave, and that is just something that has to be accepted – but if you can take time off, please do. Be a kind boss to yourself, and force yourself to look after your physical and emotional needs.

A few practical tips for returning to work:

- Prepare in your mind what you will say to work colleagues about your loss. Just having a set answer can help you deal with that unexpected conversation in the office car park.

- Try to return on a part-time basis – perhaps mornings only, or three full days – even if this is just for the first few days or weeks. A tiered return can help with the adjustment into normal life.

- Explain to your employer that on returning you may need more support, and to be met with weeks or months of backdated work will not help you perform well.

- Don't be surprised if you feel physically exhausted when you return to work. Keeping in control of your emotions is physically taxing, so add this to the daily physical tasks of your job – it makes sense why you may feel so drained.

- Ensure you have as many breaks as you are able to take. If you can take time to go for a walk, or just outside in the fresh air, do it. Take your lunch break and coffee breaks, even if you normally just power through – your mind and body will need these times to regroup.

- For the first few weeks following your return to work don't make evening plans; use your evenings to relax and process your thoughts and, importantly, to sleep. The world can quickly feel overstimulating, and you need to give your mind time each day to chill out.

- Eat healthily. The right foods can help you regain your strength and it is important to eat a balanced and healthy diet while grieving. Foods that maintain your blood glucose levels will also help you feel more emotionally stable.

The crucial thing to be aware of is that it will be hard to return to work, and the last thing you need is to be overwhelmed with work on your first week back. Be gentle with yourself and ask your employer to be thoughtful too.

> One of my greatest discoveries was that
> one cannot run out of tears.
>
> ZOË CLARK-COATES

I was really nervous of going back to work post-loss. On the one hand it felt like I should try to rejoin the world, but on the other hand it felt like a betrayal and I almost felt a little guilty. How could the world still be turning when nothing felt normal to me? How could I walk through the door of work and just slot straight back into my role, when everyone would expect the 'old' me to return? It felt a massive step. My family had suggested that I take some time off and my doctor had been willing to support this, but I also knew that for me personally, the longer I took off, the harder it would be to return to work, so I felt it best to plan a gradual return, so I could give myself time to adjust.

I had a really good boss and we arranged to meet up prior to my return to help work out the best plan of action. She helped manage some of my workload and was able to arrange for me to work remotely from home for a few days which was incredibly useful. It got me back into the swing of things while still giving me some space. She continued to check in with me over the first few weeks just to make sure that the balance was right and that I was getting the right level of support.

One of my key anxieties was breaking down at work. I was scared stiff that work colleagues would refer to my loss. Clearly, they all knew why I had been off work and I had received lots of lovely cards and messages and flowers from them in the previous weeks. I just wasn't sure that I would be able to take any face-to-face sympathetic chats or hugs from them in those first few weeks. Again, this was something my boss was able to take control of for me. She was able to let people know that, although I was immensely grateful and thankful for all their kind thoughts and messages, I just didn't want to discuss it at work and they respected that opinion and followed my wishes.

Returning to work was one of my most difficult obstacles. There were times I didn't think I would be able to get out of bed and get dressed, such was the weight of grief I felt, but I also know that work was one of my saviours. Work gave me an escape from home me. Colleagues and clients didn't know the weight of the grief baggage I was carrying, and that actually helped me. Work forced me to take some control back, and that helped me to continue to put one foot in front of the other. The first few weeks were a little blurry, if I'm honest – I was still so deep in grief and I was very hard on myself. Looking back now I recognise that I went back too soon, but it is very hard when you're in the thick of it to make truly rational decisions. I am thankful for my boss, she really did help me through, and I would encourage anyone to be as open as they can with their line manager, so they can help lead you through the first few months.

As a neonatal nurse, I love my job. It's exciting, and intense, heartbreaking at times and yet so completely fantastic when you get to see these tiny, poorly babies overcome huge hurdles to go home with their parents. Before becoming a parent, I felt I had compassion and empathy. I felt I supported my families through the hard times. I also felt I could deal with any situation, confidently and appropriately. Then we had our daughter. She was born extremely prematurely and she died within a few hours of her birth. She was with us, in our arms.

From huge excitement about being a mummy came the devastation of our loss. We had 24 hours of kindness before leaving hospital, my arms empty, and going to the nothingness that awaited us at home.

Going back to the job I loved filled me with absolute dread. Surely, every baby would remind me of mine? How could I be that confident nurse again? But every baby wasn't mine, they belonged to other desperate parents, fighting their battles with them. And I could see their fight, so raw and pure. And I had so much more insight into how I could help them. And those poor families that lose their precious babies, I could speak from the heart about the road ahead, and tell them that, while it feels like you'll never make it, one day you will remember your baby with so much love and pride and it will shape the caring and strong person you will become, because of them. I miss our daughter so much, and am often reminded of her at work, but she makes me a much stronger and better version of who I used to be.

Returning to work for me while grieving was like entering the twilight zone. I felt like a different person, but those around me assumed I would be just the same old Elle.

I sat through key business meetings trying to look composed and all together, while inside I was screaming and begging to be back home in my house, which was the only place I felt I could be real about my pain.

Anyone going through loss will know you can't control when a grief wave will hit, and that makes being at work quite scary, as it may be okay to just burst into tears in front of your family, but not so much in a meeting with all your top clients present.

However, work for me was also a good distraction; it helped me re-enter the world. It is easy to become lost in grief and almost forget who you are, but work forced me to regroup and see the world was carrying on (whether I liked that or not) and I don't think that was a bad thing.

I would say to anyone fearing returning to work to just take it a step at a time; only you know if and when you are ready to rejoin the workforce. If you do go back and then feel it was too soon, don't be afraid to say that to your boss. It's okay to step away again until you feel more ready.

SOCIAL MEDIA

Many people will tell you that they have a love-hate relationship with social media at the best of times, let alone when they are going through any traumatic or life-changing experience. My personal belief is that it can be a great tool for disseminating news and expressing feelings one may be experiencing, and it can also play a key role in bringing like-minded people together. That said, I am also acutely aware that it can make some feel very alone and judged.

The problem with social media is that if a person is seen to share 'too much' personal information they may be judged as attention-seeking. On the flipside, if a person does not share enough honest feelings, others may assume they are emotionally fine and much-needed support may not then be forthcoming. So, what is the right balance? This is something only you can determine and a lot will depend on who you are connected with on social media. If it is just family and close friends, you may feel social media is a good way to communicate your news; if you have a much wider social-media audience, you may want to be a lot more selective.

Choose whether you want to make a statement about your loss on social media. Some people want to post one message and not have to keep sharing the news, and, if you feel like this, a notice on social-media platforms may be a good option for you. Before you post your message, consider the audience, and also be clear on what you want the response to be from those who read it, maybe by including this in your post – for example, 'while we greatly value your support we would appreciate no calls for the next few days'. Practical guidance can help friends and family understand how best to respond.

Be aware that some respond on social media without properly engaging their brains, so at times people may post insensitive comments and responses. It is really hard to gauge people's intention and emotion on social media, so try to read comments and remarks with eyes of grace, and choose to think the best of people, rather than immediately taking offence. I understand this is easy to write and hard to do, but the last thing you need right now is to be carrying feelings of resentment.

If you want to keep people informed on social media but you don't feel emotionally capable, ask someone you trust to look after your accounts for a few days or weeks. They can then post your messages and respond to comments (and also delete any comments that they think you may not appreciate). Consider starting a group chat, where you can post one message to a select few family members or friends; it can be so much easier to post one message to 10 people, rather than saying the same thing over and over again.

Be aware that forums and chat rooms may not be a helpful environment for everyone. In my experience, forums and chat rooms can often bring together a lot of people who are hurting, and they can make people feel quickly lost, scared and fearing the future. Of course, there will be the exception and you may stumble across some like-minded new friends, but I always suggest one-to-one support is a lot healthier and more personal.

Follow supportive social-media accounts and pages – my Instagram and Pinterest accounts, for example, upload daily support and quotes. I do this in a bid to help people feel less alone and more understood. By sharing posts from these pages, you can also let your friends and family know how you are feeling without having to find your own words.

My top tips:

- Be cautious what you post.

- Try not to be offended if people don't respond in the way you would like, or if they don't respond at all.

- If you want specific people to know your news, ensure they do know by sending them a personal message, as it's easy to miss posts on social media, and some people who are especially close to you may feel offended to hear news about loss on social media at the same time as everyone else.

- Be prepared for people to tag you in on any story or news item they see on loss. It is often people's way of showing you they still remember what you went through.

- Most social-media platforms now allow you to mute or unfollow people's daily news and posts, and you may want to consider doing this with particular people. If hearing certain news is going to bring you any feelings of hurt or frustration, choose not to look at it; it won't help you, or help your relationship with them, so just mute their news feed (on Instagram) or unfollow their news (on Facebook). They won't ever know you have done it since you still remain as a friend and follower.

Try not to compare your grief or your story with other people's. Social media is a hothouse for this and comparing your walk through grief with another's isn't helpful or healthy. This is your walk – so, yes, be encouraged by people and use social media to feel less alone, but if someone's posts are making you feel more isolated or causing you additional pain, don't torture yourself by reading them.

> Loss has shown me so much . . . Perhaps the most important lesson of all being that I can survive even when I think I cannot.
>
> ZOË CLARK-COATES

As a self-confessed extrovert, I process the highs and lows in my life by discussing them with friends. Hairdressers. Taxi drivers. Total strangers. We encountered loss while taking a year out travelling around the world, and I decided to share our utter heartbreak on Instagram. I was posting a daily travel caption anyway, and it felt right to share about this too.

I poured my heart out to my online friends, sharing the pain that I was feeling and acknowledging that I probably wasn't alone – chances were some people reading it would have experienced the same pain. What I didn't expect were the 700 messages and comments I received.

All of them supportive, and most of them – sadly – with a personal understanding of loss. Social media can get a bad rap but, in the most painful period of our lives, my husband and I found it nothing but a buoyancy aid. We clung to each other: talking till our voices were hoarse, dancing in the garden to music only we could hear, and crying hot, bitter tears. Then, when we needed to look outside of ourselves, we read messages from strangers. They were so comforting. There is something beautifully infectious about honesty. So, for me, sharing was a good thing, a beautiful thing, and I have no regrets in doing it.

SPECIAL AND NOTABLE OCCASIONS

Until you have lived a full year following the loss of your loved one, you have no idea what may become a key trigger (and even after that 12-month milestone new triggers can appear). There are, of course, key occasions to be aware of which may (and probably will) cause new grief layers to be pulled back. These are:

- Birthdays
- Anniversaries
- Due dates
- Mother's and Father's Day
- Loss or Charity Awareness Weeks
- Christmas and other widely celebrated holidays and occasions

I call the moments of grief that hit us from nowhere and bring us to our knees 'grief thunderbolts', and if we try to predict and pre-empt what may or may not cause them, we can become constantly fearful of the future. The bottom line is it is impossible to envisage when they might strike. Even unrelated deaths, events or occasions can trigger waves of grief, as anything that taps into similar emotions can initiate a fresh wave to hit. We just have to bravely move forwards and deal with our reaction whenever and wherever these thunderbolts do strike us down.

Facing our grief is daring and it's bold; it takes real courage – looking loss directly in the eye and still choosing to steadily move towards it. We have to face these key occasions, whether we feel ready or not.

What I can say to you to hopefully bring you some reassurance is this: 90 per cent of the time the fear of the event is much worse than the reality of actually walking through the occasion, so try going into events and key dates with an open mind and without preconceptions of how you 'may' feel. Just say to yourself, whatever I feel is okay. If I cry – that is okay. If another grief layer is harshly pulled off – that is fine. If I feel absolutely nothing – that is equally fine.

Some people choose to mark occasions by doing something special; others prefer to carry on as normal. I encourage you to do whatever you feel is right for you and your family. Remember, this is your journey, your story – you write the rule book.

If you are looking for ideas, here are a few things that I know can help:

- Light a candle on special days
- Hang a Christmas decoration on the tree each year with your loved one's name on it
- Plant a tree or plant
- Donate money or time to a charity or cause in honour of your loved one
- Carry out random acts of kindness in honour of your loved one
- Visit a special place
- Read a special book which makes you feel connected to the person you have lost

Occasions and events can encourage us to be more vulnerable, as we are often forced or persuaded to share our pain and stories with those around us. This in turn helps those who care for us, as they can better understand the pain that is being carried by their loved one (it also often gives them permission to share any pain and grief they may personally be carrying).

One of my favourite C. S. Lewis quotes is from his book *The Four Loves*. He wrote so eloquently about grief.

> *To love at all is to be vulnerable. Love anything and your heart will be wrung and possibly broken.*
>
> *If you want to make sure of keeping it intact you must give it to no one, not even an animal. Wrap it carefully round with hobbies and little luxuries; avoid all entanglements. Lock it up safe in the casket or coffin of your selfishness. But in that casket, safe, dark, motionless, airless, it will change. It will not be broken; it will become unbreakable, impenetrable, irredeemable. To love is to be vulnerable.*

So let me encourage you to choose courage. To bravely reject society's often subtle message to deny one's grief and pain, in a bid not to disturb a happy equilibrium. Be vulnerable, however hard that may seem, as the more open you are, the more you will feel connected to those around you.

4
Post-loss

SUPPORTING THE BEREAVED

There are so many ways we can all help the bereaved, and what I would love this book to do is empower you to reach out with confidence to someone who is grieving. The fact that you are even trying to educate yourself on this subject and are researching how best to support someone means *you* are the right person for the job. You want to be the best support you can be, and that makes you one amazing person, so I want to thank you for taking the time to learn about this complex subject.

When I went through loss, I so appreciated those who offered me a hand of support. Some people took to supporting me like a duck to water; others were visibly treading water and were trying to look like they could swim. I appreciated each and every one of them. Those who said amazing things, those who stumbled over their words, and even those who said things that really shouldn't have been said. I loved that they tried; I appreciated that they cared enough to sit with me, even if they didn't feel comfortable doing so. So please don't be worried; just be there whenever they need you, love them, sprinkle kindness on them and be willing to step outside of your comfort zone.

Now, I'm going to warn you that some of my suggestions may seem quite forthright. I never want people to feel told off, or judged, or panicked, but I do want you to feel fully informed. I want to equip you with the right empathy tools, and the best way to do that is to tell you some commonly said things that can cause offence, and also some good things to say that can bring comfort.

It would be easy for me to tiptoe around this, but that won't help you, or help the people you want to support, so I am going to be direct and say it how it is in the hope you can receive it in love.

If you read something in the 'do not say this' section and you have said it, please don't panic. I don't want anyone to feel shame or guilt. All of us can and will have said the wrong things, me included (probably many times a day!), so don't beat yourself up. Instead, say, 'Okay, I will know what to say next time.' If you feel you may have caused unintentional pain to someone in the past, you may, of course, want to address that, and I would purely suggest saying something along the lines of this: 'Having read *Beyond Goodbye* I have learnt I may have said some insensitive things in the past. I trust you know my heart has only ever been to help you, but if I ever caused you additional pain, I am so sorry. I now feel better equipped to support you and others, and please always feel free to tell me if I say anything wrong in the future.' Saying something as simple as this is the ultimate olive branch, and can bring so much healing to unhealed wounds.

My best advice

Don't compare

Every journey is unique; therefore, even if you have been through something similar it will be different from the person in front of you, so don't rush to share your story about grief or loss, or say, 'This is how I felt, do you?'

Let them tell you their story first in their own words. By doing this the attention will also be kept on the person who's hurting, rather than transferring to you. If you have lost your partner and they have lost their partner, your stories may have significant similarities, but your journey through grief will be surprisingly different. Once they have shared, then open up about your story if you feel able.

One of my most precious times when I was at the rawest point of grief was when a friend sat on my bed and shared her experience of loss; it did make me feel less alone, so choose your words carefully and pick your moment wisely.

Be present

When researching this book, I asked people about the things said to them that caused pain. Perhaps not surprisingly, I received a long list, but one of the things that most people agreed on was that being there, and showing up, even if at times the wrong things were said, mattered more to them.

Having people avoid you, or avoid the topic of loss, causes way more pain than stumbling with words, or being a tad insensitive. So be brave and show up, however uncomfortable it makes you feel. Remember, you don't need to say anything; just hold the tissues, and tell them you care and want to listen.

Accept you can't fix it

Part of showing up and being present for the grieving is having to accept that you can't fix it for the person. Everything within you will want to make it better for them, as human instinct is to try to relieve another's suffering, but that's not possible when it comes to grief.

If you see it as your job to fix it, or to remove it, then, of course, very quickly you will feel overwhelmed in your task of offering support, as it is an impossible job and the goal will never be achieved. You will then begin to feel helpless and may start to panic; you may even want to run for cover as it could feel too hard to be that shoulder to cry on.

To avoid this happening, be aware that you will have an urge to fix it, but choose to accept that you can't. This acceptance will give you the freedom to just be you; you will realise that all you have the power to do is to listen, to offer support without judgement and without providing temporary fixes, and I promise you this will be a gift to the person who is grieving.

Never minimise

When we are supporting the bereaved, we need to be careful never to minimise their grief, or oversimplify the walk through loss. I would recommend not to start a sentence with 'at least', as 99 per cent of the time that will be a form of minimising a person's pain – for example, 'At least they aren't in pain anymore', 'At least you can focus on you now', 'At least you have your sibling to help you', etc.

There is *no* 'at least' in grief support.

Be aware of what they have lost

It is easy to forget that when people lose someone, they aren't just losing them at the age at which they died. They are also losing their birthday each year. They are missing that key event the whole family were looking forward to. They are missing the holiday they always go on together. Plus a million other life events. In the blink of an eye, the future has been erased.

Remembering this transforms how we offer support to the bereaved, as you become aware of why the journey through grief does actually take a lifetime. The person will be mourning another stage of loss, another moment stolen from them, until the day they die.

Frequently asked questions

Can you move on following loss?

I often witness people talking about those who are grieving. Some of the most common comments appear to be: 'They seem to be stuck in grief' or 'They just haven't been able to move on'. These statements are used whenever a period of time has passed since the death of the loved one and the person is still talking about the loss, or showing visible signs of grief.

Firstly, grief and loss are not something you 'get over',

so just because someone is talking about the loss still, or is displaying symptoms of grief, this in no way means they are 'stuck'; it merely means they are processing, and that could be something they do for the rest of their life.

The loss of a loved one becomes part of who you are, and you learn to carry the weight of the grief and allow it to shape you into a different person.

How can we help people get to this stage in their grief journey?

By allowing them space to talk and share. If we try to rush people to process pain, it has the reverse effect and sets them back in their walk, so all we can do is walk alongside them and hopefully you will then start to witness them rediscovering their joy.

Can you become stuck in grief?

People often come to me saying their family member or friend is stuck in grief, and how can we help them as a charity.

My first question is what do you mean by 'stuck'? Just because someone is talking about the person they have lost, it does not mean they are stuck. Just because someone is still weeping and heartbroken, it does not mean they are stuck.

That is how grief works; they are meant to still talk about their loss, and they are grieving healthily if they still communicate about the one they have lost.

My worry is for the person who can't talk about their pain, and for the one who makes it seem like no loss has even happened.

So, is it possible to get stuck in grief?

Yes, I believe it is. I would question (and notice I say question, not assume) whether someone was stuck if their loss was a long time ago but they were still finding it impossible to talk about anything other than their pain.

I would also consider whether someone was stuck if (after a substantial amount of time) they felt it impossible to move forwards in ordinary life because of being consumed by sorrow. However, that said, there are no set rules and no set formulas when it comes to moving through the grieving process. One plus one doesn't always equal two when it comes to grief.

What can we do if we think someone is stuck?

There is only one thing anyone can do and that is listen to their story.

Hear their pain.

Validate their experience.

Show you care.

People mostly get stuck because they are feeling a need to defend their right to be experiencing pain, as they don't feel their story is being heard. They may also feel the need to ensure their loved one is being acknowledged and not forgotten. Simply by listening, we can help them unstick themselves.

Can you get closure?

Closure following a loss is as much of a myth as unicorns and fairy tales. You cannot close the door on grief. It is just not possible to put all feelings into a box, seal the lid and consider it part of the past.

You can only learn to accept what has happened and learn to live with this new state of reality. Compartmentalising feelings invariably leads to unresolved grief bubbling through at another time in a person's life, often negatively affecting their physical, emotional or mental well-being.

Does publicly grieving help?

Public grieving helps because we can suddenly see we are not alone in our pain. There is a reason we hold funerals, there is a reason that people around the world gather to remember and celebrate the lives of those who have died, and that reason is that something powerful happens when we stand together. We feel supported. We feel less alone. We feel our loved one has been duly honoured. We feel our pain and loss have been recognised. Seeing all of this and exploring all of this helps hearts begin to mend.

One of the most vital things the Mariposa Trust does is run the international 'Saying Goodbye' services of remembrance. These public events are held at cathedrals all over the world, and they allow people from every generation a time and place to publicly grieve and acknowledge every baby they or someone else has lost.

The services aren't about 'closure', they aren't an opportunity for people to formally say goodbye so they can 'move on'; they are about healing the pain, acknowledging a baby existed, honouring the love that did and will always exist and giving space for people to say publicly, 'My child matters.'

How do you know if someone is depressed or grieving?

You won't know this, and often the bereaved person may not even know it. I will always look for signs of depression in a person if they have suffered from depression pre-loss. Grief tends to come in waves; depression doesn't move, it stays like a black cloud. Grief can trigger depression. Grief can develop into depression. However, mostly grief stays as grief and is not 'depression' at all.

Be careful with how you word questions about how they are feeling and encourage them to share their worries and concerns. GPs are trained to help people determine whether they are depressed, so I would always encourage a person to sit with a doctor and talk about their feelings and symptoms, and then the doctor can advise them on what is best to do next.

A big alarm bell for me would be talk or mention of suicide. There is a *big* difference between someone not wanting to live (because of the depth of the pain they are experiencing and the overwhelming feelings of missing the person they have lost) and being suicidal. It is very common not to want to be here anymore – who would want to live in agony daily and see no chance of respite on the horizon? Being suicidal is very different and if someone is considering ending their life or you feel he or she is at risk of this, encourage them to seek urgent medical help.

Things not to say and why

I am regularly asked by people and the media what you shouldn't say. I prefer to focus on the right things to say, but I can also see a real benefit in highlighting the pitfalls and the things that are habitually voiced to the bereaved.

So here goes – buckle up, my friends, and let me take you on a journey of clichés and the reasons why they cause pain.

'Let go'

If you say to someone, 'Let go of the pain' or 'You need to let go of your loved one now and just move on', you will be causing deep hurt, and I know that is the last thing you would want to do.

It's not possible to 'let go' of someone you have loved and lost, emotion doesn't work like that. In fact, love doesn't work like that. Although someone is no longer living life with a person in the physical sense, the love for them is acutely present. The only thing they need you to do is walk with them, help them to carry the load any way you can, journey with them as they learn to juggle the mammoth task of processing grief and pain while remaining present in the world.

'Perhaps they died due to x/y/z?'

This guessing doesn't help anyone, and even though you are trying to find a reason in your mind why someone may have died, so that it makes sense to you, it helps no one and brings more pain to the person who is grieving.

'It is time to move on/get over it/stop talking about it!'

Grief is not something one gets over, and talking about the pain of loss is the best way for people to start to heal, so this needs to be encouraged and never discouraged.

'God didn't want them to stay'/'They are in a better place now they are in heaven'

This is just so painful and insensitive.

Avoid bringing God into the conversation, as, whether or not a person has faith, God didn't make this happen and trying to insinuate that their loved one is in a better place says their home on earth was not the best place for them, which is hurtful.

'Time will heal your pain'/'Life goes on'

Yes, at times pain can decrease over time; however, it can also increase. No bereaved person will thank you for telling them that life will get better down the line, while they are in the depths of grief, so avoid telling them it will.

Just let them focus on today, as that can seem daunting enough when you are journeying through loss.

'At least they lived until they were a good age'

Another 'at least', so we know it shouldn't be said at all. Sadly, this is said so often to people who lose an elderly partner, parent or grandparent. Just because someone is older doesn't make the pain and grief any less important.

'At least they are out of pain'

As above . . . But again, this is so commonly said to people, especially if the person who has died suffered from any sort of disease or condition that meant they experienced acute pain.

No one wants to see their loved one suffering, and, yes, you would be right to think this is possibly one of the only positive outcomes following the death of someone who was in agony, but it actually doesn't help to be reminded of it many times a day when grieving. If the bereaved person is saying it, that is of course totally fine. However, it's often said to try to make a person look on the bright side, and it's much better to let them process the grief they are carrying.

'You are lucky you already have children/siblings etc.'

Of course, every child is a real blessing, but having children or other siblings doesn't remove the grief you feel for the child/sibling you have lost. Let's imagine a situation where you have two children, and I turn to you and say, 'Which of your children are you willing to lose? You can only keep one of them!' You would never be able to answer and neither should you, yet when a bereaved parent loses a child, or a sibling loses a brother or sister, often people expect them to be grateful for the one (or more) they still have with them. It is bizarre and insulting.

'You are blessed you have your health'

This is another 'let's search for a blessing' ideology, in the hope it will negate the pain. It doesn't work; let's not do it.

'This is super-common, you know'

Yes, loss is common; however, that does not make it less painful, or something anyone should expect.

'Because you have been through it before, you can cope again'

Just because someone has survived one loss, it does not automatically make them better equipped to deal with it a second, third or fourth time.

Yes, a loss may have taught them some valuable life lessons or coping skills, but this can never be presumed, and should certainly never be spoken out loud. Every loss is different, and personality, life circumstances, emotional stability, physical health, etc. all play a part in how people cope.

'What doesn't kill you makes you stronger'

Let's avoid this commonly voiced cliché.

'Once you have another child/partner your pain will go'

Entirely untrue, and no bereaved parent or widow/widower would ever agree. It should never be thought or communicated. Another person will never replace the one who has died, and while other people are an absolute gift and blessing, their presence doesn't take away the pain of losing the person who has died.

'In other countries, people expect to lose people from that; it's only here we don't'

This may be true, but showing someone how privileged we are to live in this country doesn't help their pain. You are just subtly (or possibly not so subtly) removing their permission to grieve.

'My friend lost their x when they died from y – that is much worse, isn't it?'

Comparison helps no one. There is no score attributable to grief and loss. Why does one have to be worse than another? Instead, let's stand together and say all loss is horrid, every death is traumatic, and every person touched by loss deserves to and should be supported.

'Do you think they died due to a genetic issue or hereditary illness?'

Who knows, and is it up to you to ask? This is a highly personal question and not one to be asked by someone who is trying to offer valuable support.

'Have you heard about this study or x/y/z information – it may help you find a reason for the death?'

I know this comes from a real wish to help, but sadly it's often not taken in that way, and could be seen as, 'If you had known about x/y/z, your loved one wouldn't have died.'

'It's good that they died quickly and didn't suffer as long as x!'

Another statement that minimises someone's loss and grief. The length of an illness doesn't change the amount someone grieves.

'I am sure you will meet someone else!'

Many who lose a partner don't want to meet another person and hearing such statements while they are grieving can be utterly heartbreaking. Let's not focus on further relationships; let's focus all attention on the person they have lost.

'In a few weeks, you will be like a whole new person!'

Positivity doesn't change the reality, and while you might like to fast-forward time so that the person standing in front of you isn't in pain, you cannot rescue them, and you can't say with all honesty that things will be better soon. By even trying to do this you remove yourself from being a trusted and reliable confidante, as it shows a real lack of empathy and compassion to speak with such authority about something you have no actual knowledge of.

'Maybe if you didn't think about it, it would be easier'

Grief can't be denied or avoided. In fact, the more you try not to think about it, the more it can overwhelm the brain. It needs time and space to be processed, so by encouraging people not to think about the loss, you are doing them a disservice.

'Perhaps you are dwelling on it too much'

While it is possible to get overly consumed with focusing on loss (which of course wouldn't be healthy), the majority of people aren't dwelling on grief; they are simply trying to survive the loss. Their brain needs time to come to terms with the trauma, and unless they give themselves space to focus on their situation, they will never be able to move forwards healthily. Let me also remind you that there is no 'normal' when it comes to loss, so who can even determine what is 'too much'? Too much to you may not be enough for another person, so we must be mindful not to judge or critique how any person journeys through grief.

'Maybe this is just a sign that you shouldn't be a parent or aren't ready to be a parent'

It is hard to believe that this is ever said to a grieving parent, but I have heard it being uttered, so I know it happens. It's often said to teenage mums, where people feel they have almost been rescued from an unplanned pregnancy, but I have also heard of it being told to parents who have encountered large numbers of miscarriages. It is hurtful, it's thoughtless and should never be thought, let alone voiced.

'Aren't you feeling better yet?'

Usually, this question gets asked within two to four weeks of a funeral – shocking, isn't it? Sadly, if people don't grieve fast enough, the world often makes them feel abnormal for still hurting, for still crying and for still feeling broken. As soon as you say the words 'aren't you', you are putting an expectation on that person, that they should be further on in their journey, and that brings more hurt and pain to their door. Instead, ask: 'How are you feeling today?' Or: 'Have you been able to experience any moments of peace this week?'

'When do you think you will be back to normal?'

I can answer this one for you. Never. People who have experienced loss never return to the old them.

Loss and grief change you forever, so if you can accept that and then gently help the bereaved person discover it, you will be an excellent support for them as they walk through grief.

As long as the sun continues to shine,
and the stars light up the darkest of skies,
I will miss you

ZOË CLARK-COATES
the babylossguide.com

PROACTIVE ADVICE FOR FAMILY AND FRIENDS

Having covered what not to say, I would love now to offer you some practical tips on how you can support someone who has lost a loved one. Prior to being trained and then subsequently working in the field of bereavement care, I remember feeling so confused when I was faced with helping bereaved friends and family members – I wanted to make things better for them, but I didn't know what help to offer. I hope this chapter makes you feel empowered and equipped to support any broken-hearted people on your path through life.

When supporting a loved one, you need to realise that things can stack up and suddenly reach crisis point, so be aware of some of the typical responses:

Wanting to run away: What they want is to escape the pain, and, in their head, they feel like they can run away from it. Unfortunately, this is not the case, and even if they do travel, the grief goes with them. Listen to them expressing their heart's desire.

Not wanting to leave the house: Often people find security in their home and can almost become phobic about leaving their house, as the world can feel like a terrifying place. Of course, I would not advocate dragging people outside against their will, but I do always recommend gently encouraging people to step out their front door regularly. The longer it is left, the harder it can become to do. Little and often is a right approach.

Panic attacks: Some may have experienced these pre-loss, but for others the loss may have triggered their first attack; either way, it is terrifying for the person. Be aware that this isn't something that can just be brushed off and it is the brain's way of saying, 'I can't cope right now.' Gently encourage them to seek help from a professional and chat with their GP.

Lack of appetite/eating much more than usual: Most of the time, people's appetite will return to normal within a month, so encourage them to take plenty of fluids.

Eating little and often is usually more comfortable for those in the depths of grief, and a great gift is lots of snack packs, as nibbling on food can make appetite return. If their regular eating pattern doesn't resume within a month, I will often suggest a person should sit down and talk in depth with a friend or a professional, to see if verbalising their grief helps.

What to consider

Please don't be scared about seeing pain and grief up close and personal. Yes, it is hard to see someone you care about upset, but if you were in their shoes you would want the people you love to surround you, and you can be one of these people to them.

- Be aware that grief can trigger a host of other emotional issues. If someone has issues in his or her marriage/relationship, they are likely to surface at this time. Similarly, if a person has issues with their parents or siblings, these are likely to come to a breaking point at this time of emotional crisis.

- Seek to understand more about loss and grief if you haven't personally experienced it. It is easy to oversimplify loss and almost consider it unnatural, but it is one of the most natural parts of life; there is a time to be born and a time to die. If you can become comfortable talking about the subject of death, you will be able to support the grieving much better.

- Don't presume anger is part of grief. Of course, some people may experience a degree of anger in the grieving process; however, many won't, and to assume someone's anger is just part of grief can be harmful to the individual and mean injustices aren't addressed.

- Think before you share. When you are bereaved, some information is more painful to hear. For example, 'I can't believe my husband is constantly coming in late from work, can you?' This can be a kick in the guts to someone who has just lost their partner, so be aware of this. Grief can make people less patient for a time and also blunter, so think and be mindful. This doesn't mean you shouldn't share about your life at all. I welcomed news of other life issues or situations when I was grieving; it gave me time to think of someone else, but how it was shared was significant.

- Know and accept they are likely to be tired most of the time. Grief is exhausting; it uses every bit of the physical and mental energy available to a person, and often that means they spend a lot of their time saying how tired they are. Reassure them that it is normal, and when you see them or do activities together, perhaps focus on things that don't need much physical energy.

- Often bereaved people will tell you they forget things all the time and find it difficult to focus; this is just because their brain is in overdrive dealing with the pain of loss. Think of it like a computer having a hundred tabs open on the browser – everything slows down, and sometimes the whole PC needs to shut down and reboot. Offer gentle reminders to those you are supporting to alleviate the pressure, even if it's just by sending a simple text – for instance, 'Looking forward to seeing you tomorrow at 1pm.' Then you aren't highlighting the fact they may not have remembered the arrangement or the time.

- It is okay to laugh and smile. One of the things that the bereaved struggle with is allowing themselves to smile without feeling guilty, as they fear those around them will assume they are 'over the loss' if they laugh. It can also feel disloyal to the person they have lost to smile and enjoy life. I spend my life reassuring the bereaved that it's not only okay to smile, but it's also crucial that they do, as the brain can only handle so much trauma, and it needs light relief and an escape at times.

- Children and babies (post someone losing a child). For some, children are hard to be around post-loss, for others (and I fell into this category) they bring them hope and relief. Every time I saw a baby, a child or even a pregnancy bump I thought, it can go well for me as it did/has for them – they were like rays of hope wherever I looked. For others it brings pain, and every pregnancy bump they see feels like a slap in the face. The only person who can tell you how they feel is the bereaved person, so ask them. Let them set the agenda here; if they prefer only to see non-pregnant people or babies for a time, that is their choice. Nothing you say will change how they feel, so even if you disagree with how they may handle it, be kind, gentle and non-judgemental. Whatever helps them survive their journey of loss is a good thing – remember that!

What to say

Remember, showing up is ultimately what matters. Don't be so afraid of saying the wrong thing that you hide away and say nothing at all. I would much rather have someone say something than someone who ignores my suffering.

- Let the bereaved set the tone and the agenda rather than presuming. Let them say if they feel happy, sad, confused or lost. If they control the dialogue, it ensures what you say is appropriate to how they feel in that moment.

- Ask in-depth questions, not just surface ones.

It is easy to stick to 'safe' questions; for example, 'How are you doing?' However, most of the time people will have become so practised at answering these that they answer before they even think, and will reply, 'Coping, thanks' or, 'I'm okay, thanks.' By just going a little broader, and reframing questions, you can properly engage with people who need to talk about their pain.

How about asking:

- 'What was your most difficult moment to navigate this week?'

- 'Did you find joy in anything this week?'
- 'Was there anything you needed this week that I could have helped you with?'

Pay close attention to their response. If they respond openly, that's great. If they don't, spend time thinking about how better to phrase a question for the next time you see them. Prior preparation can make you feel more confident in your interaction, and once you have truly engaged them in conversation, you won't need to say much as the bereaved person will do most of the talking.

- Ask questions about their experience of loss. People are often desperate to share their stories (even if they do shed copious amounts of tears in the process). Of course, some of these may be hard to hear, but some will also be beautiful.

Believe me when I say that every time you sit and listen to a bereaved person's story, you are giving them a real gift.

What to do

Most people will rush to support those grieving in the couple of weeks immediately following a loss, but this often then dwindles or stops altogether. People naturally go back to their typical day-to-day lives and presume the bereaved person has moved on too. But they won't have; they are just as heartbroken, and are often now left with little or no support. Be aware of this and increase your support in the weeks that follow, rather than reducing it.

- Ensure they have details of the support available to them. People have to want support, and reaching out for it is the first part of their healing process.

- Do things that show the bereaved person you are thinking of them, even if you can't see them face to face (at all or daily/weekly). Send them notes, text messages, cards, gifts. A book can be a helpful gift so that, if and when they feel they need help or assistance, it will already be at their fingertips.

- Make a note in your diary of key anniversaries and reach out to the bereaved in the weeks before the date to say, 'I am thinking of you, leading up to x anniversary' – this means the world to grieving people. Then also reach out to them on the day, even if you only send a card. Then it is just as important to contact them a few weeks after and ask them how they coped.

- Offer practical help at home. Try to be more specific than saying, 'Call me if you need help.' Instead try: 'Are you okay with me bringing dinner over for the next few weeks?' Or, 'Can I stock your freezer with ready-made meals so that when you have no desire to cook or even eat, there is food there for you?' Or, 'Can I come and vacuum, clean or do your ironing?'

When someone is struggling to survive the weight of grief, household chores are the last thing on their mind, and if you can help make their living environment a nicer or tidier space, that is a gift. When you spend a lot of time crying on the bathroom floor, it being clean is a blessing.

- If the bereaved person has children, offer to help take care of them. While it is good for children to see that grief and loss are part of life, and that crying is okay and indeed healthy, they also have a limit on how much they can tolerate. If you can take them out, and allow them to have times of fun and joy amid the sorrow, that can be helpful for the parents.

- Offer physical touch if appropriate. Now, this comes with a warning, as some people hate physical touch and will avoid it at all costs, so only make physical contact if you know the person well enough to be sure they will welcome it.

Touch is important when offering compassion and empathy because it can make people feel heard and loved. Just holding their hand or hugging them can make them feel safer, grounded and cared for.

- Arrange meetings/hang-outs where they will feel at ease being real. Many people aren't naturally comfortable at dinner parties at the best of times, and events like this are even harder when you feel bereft, so try to create more casual and relaxed opportunities, so they don't feel a need to put on a 'brave face'. Please also be mindful of holding more formal events and not inviting the bereaved person, as that can cause real hurt. So, yes, you may need to change how you do things for a few months, but if it helps the grieving person, surely it's worth it?

- Be flexible with plans. Make it clear you are fine if the arrangements change right up to the last minute. Often what stops people who are grieving making plans is that they are worried they may suddenly not feel able to go out, which means it feels safer to them not to make any arrangements with anyone for fear of letting others down. By giving them permission always to change, cancel or move events, you will provide them with the peace of mind they need to take the risk.

If/when the person does change arrangements, be sure never to make them feel guilty or to look put out, even if you have to do a fantastic acting job. (Yes, I know you are human too, so may feel disappointed if the day at the spa is cancelled an hour before you were due to leave, hence my acting suggestion . . .)

- Be forgiving and patient. When journeying through grief, it can mean a person feels so overwhelmed and numb that they stop being thoughtful or kind. They may appear emotionless or too emotional. They may be brutal in their responses and lack sensitivity in how they phrase things.

They may not ask how your day went or for news on your work promotion.

I urge you to accept that this isn't personal, and it does not mean the bereaved person has become selfish and self-centred. It just says they are crawling through life right now, and they are so overwhelmed with pain, their typical responses to things are on hold. Give them time, and they will start asking about you again; it won't always be about them.

Support for the supporters

I think we need to discuss another tier of support that I never hear being talked about and that is support for those who are doing the supporting. We all talk about the first line of support, those who are sitting with the bereaved, or those who are nursing the dying, but we don't often discuss supporting the supporters.

I think it's easy to fall into a pattern of saying to these people, 'Don't forget about looking after you too', 'Don't take on too much' or 'Remember you also need space', but actually this can add to the pressure. When you are offering vital support, the needs of the supporter will automatically (and probably rightly) take second place, but carrying the stress and grief, as well as providing the practical support, can be utterly exhausting. I know that no matter how many times people said to me, 'Make sure you take time for you, Zoë', it went in one ear and out the other, as, however nice a concept this was, I was aware I had no choice but to keep showing up and offering the support that was required.

So how can people help? Well, perhaps change the dialogue. Instead of coming out with clichés, ask direct and thoughtful questions, like: 'What was your toughest moment today?' Or: 'Did you feel supported today?' Real questions that open the conversation and allow the person to share their feelings.

Send them funny things to read, or thoughtful cards, to show them their compassion is being honoured and not overlooked.

(Remember, the bereaved or the dying will often not be in a position to commend and applaud, and you being that voice can really encourage someone to keep going.)

Send them flowers to cheer them along and offer them practical support, such as cooking them meals. If they are spending all their time caring for others, they are probably not finding much time to prepare their own dinner.

So, the bottom line is this: If you aren't required to be the support-giver, please be the supporter's support and cheerleader, as that is also helping the bereaved or the dying via another route.

Following gathering the pieces of their broken heart up off the floor, there is another epic mountain bereaved people have to attempt to climb, and that is learning to live again. Their lives have been about surviving, about creating defence strategies to protect their aching hearts, and then the world tells them it's time to re-engage with society . . . and believe me it is not that simple. It's an Everest-sized task. So reach out, show love, compassion and offer a helping hand – carry their bag, secure their harness, and most importantly become their companion on the journey.

ZOË CLARK-COATES

5

Layers of Grief

You may have read many articles and leaflets on grief and loss, which allude to the fact that there are set stages. These are usually:

- Denial
- Anger
- Bargaining
- Depression
- Acceptance

While these can be accurate for some, those who go through grief via these steps, in this set order, will definitely be in the minority. Grief is not that straightforward. It may be easier to talk about myself when explaining this. Once I was told about the loss of our baby, I didn't go into denial. I never felt any anger about their death, not anger at myself or the hospital, or my family – none, no anger at all. I then didn't bargain. I didn't have depression. However, I did get acceptance. I would say my stages of grief looked more like this.

- Shocked
- Scared
- Shocked
- Confused
- Lost
- Acceptance

Every person's steps will be unique to them, even if there are strong common themes or similarities with those of others.

Grief really can come off in layers – one minute you can be fine and the next you are crying, and this can happen over years or even over a lifetime. Society tells us everything has a time limit, and that is a strongly held belief when it comes to grief. The sad part of this is that it means most people grieve in silence. This is especially true if a person didn't feel able to process their grief at the time of their loss. If years later they allow themselves time to process the pain, society often doesn't respect and acknowledge how vital this is to a person's well-being, and can make them feel shame for expressing their pain and sadness so long after the loss has happened.

When we launched the Mariposa Trust and the Saying Goodbye Remembrance Services, we initially thought they would be for recently bereaved people, but we were so wrong. They have been happening now for many years, and every single service is made up of people who have lost recently, as well as those who lost their children 40, 50, 60, 70 years ago. Many people in their eighties and nineties attend who recount their inability to grieve at the time of their loss or losses; they explain how they have carried their grief for decades, and how finally coming to a service has allowed them to openly express their pain and grief.

Grief is a long journey; it will be patient and travel with a person until they are ready or able to process it.

One extra note of caution is this: Once you have survived a significant loss you are forever changed. I believe one of the ramifications of this is that, if you lose other people you love in the future, you will never again grieve only for the person who has just died, you will recommence grieving for all the people you have loved and lost. This can make future losses more challenging, and you may quickly feel consumed with grief. Please try not to be scared and simply allow yourself to face the pain, and deal with the many grief layers that are being internally processed.

A short while ago, I was talking to my friend one evening and she was telling me how she couldn't stop crying and how her grief for the children she had lost many years ago suddenly felt fresh and raw again.

This new layer of grief was triggered by her youngest son leaving for university. Nothing could have prepared her for this wave to hit, as she had never lived through the experience of suddenly having no children residing at home. I asked Siobhan if she could explain the pain, and this is what she said.

Sometimes we are simply not ready for a new grief layer to be revealed. One moment you are enjoying life, the next you are wailing on the floor begging for this gut wrenching pain to end. I wonder if it's griefs way of asserting its power, ensuring we know that she is in charge and not us.

ZOË CLARK-COATES

It took me 10 pregnancies to get my three sons. The miscarriages ranged from early- to late-gestation losses and each of the losses threads through my very being. I have got to the stage of my grief where I have accepted the losses and use my experience to help others in my daily work. Or so I thought.

If my last losses had survived the pregnancies, my children would now be 15, 14 and 11. My youngest live son is 18 and I proudly sent him off to university in September, the third of the brothers to go in three years. As his survival was a miracle and he nearly died at birth due to my blood-clotting disorder, the pride is even more enormous at his achievement.

The joy I feel at how well my three sons are all doing at university is accentuated each day when we chat on the phone about how their day has been. So the ferocity of the 'empty-nest syndrome' was unexpected to say the least. I miss my boys, but it was so much more than that. The truth is that my home should not be child-free; it should still have children here if they had not died, and this grief is overwhelming. I feel that I have lost them all over again and that grief is raw and painful.

Maybe having live children tempered the grief I experienced through all the losses and what I am experiencing now is more real.

Although what I feel now seems sadly familiar – the tears, physical heartache, the nightmares and waking up crying and shouting out are things I thought I had left behind.

I find myself imagining my lost children in the empty spaces left by their university-student brothers.

So I don't know how to cope with this grief, as although it feels familiar I am struggling with finding a way out of it due to the unexpectedness of it all. I feel I am back to square one, but this time there is one crucial difference. I know I have a support system around me who understand the grief and I am now not alone as a grieving mother.

These layers can be revealed at any time, and you can't prepare for it; all you can do is not be scared of it when it shows its face. If you don't fight it, or resist processing the pain that surfaces, the tears will settle, and the grief will quickly soften again so it becomes easier to carry. Grief is like an onion made up of many, many layers. These layers of 'grief' can be exposed at any moment.

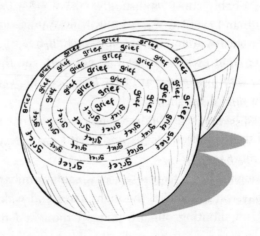

HEALING

This is a difficult subject to explore but I know I need to include it in this book as I am asked about it constantly. 'Do people heal post-loss?' The answer is some do, and some don't.

In order to explain this, let's put the spotlight on me and talk about my personal experience of child loss . . .

Firstly, I guess we need to decipher what I mean by 'heal'. To me, not healing means someone feels: Despair. Hopelessness. Physical and mental torture about the loss. Being constantly unhappy.

I don't feel those things anymore, which is why I feel my heart has healed. I fully accept I have children who didn't survive, and I have come to terms with the pain of losing them. There will always be parts of me missing, as I have five little ones not sitting here in my home, and that will never be 'okay', but I also feel blessed that they were here at all. Probably, most importantly, I have gone on to be happier than I ever was pre-loss in their honour.

Will I always talk about them? *YES! They are as much my children as my living children here with me are, so of course I will talk about them, celebrate them and smile when I think about them.*

Do I miss them? *Yes, desperately.*

Do I wish they hadn't died? *Yes, of course, I long for them to be here with me.*

Do I have times where grief can hit me out of nowhere and I have a cry? *Yes! Very rarely, but I still have those times.*

Does it hurt to talk about the children I lost? *No, not at all. I love talking about all my children, and the experience of losing them is now part of my story and I feel totally comfortable talking about every detail of it.*

So why do some people not heal following losing a loved one? This is pretty impossible to answer, as everyone is unique, but I think I can unravel some of the myths surrounding it.

If someone doesn't heal, does it mean they loved the person they have lost more than someone else whose heart has healed? No, of course it doesn't. Love and healing aren't linked.

The reason I knew I needed to address this in my book is that so many people ask me every week how I have found a path of total joy to walk down, following loss. They want to know how they can experience the same, and how they can use the grief they have experienced to embrace life more. The reason I have shared my story publicly is to try to bring hope to people who are desperate, to be a light when people are crawling around in the dark, and I would never want anyone to think that as soon as they lose a loved one they are doomed to an unhappy life, as it's not always like that for everyone.

I would like to say that having a healed heart does not mean that people won't at times feel broken, or feel acute pain, or feel grief-stricken and freshly bereaved. This is sadly part of grief and the walk of grief takes a lifetime.

Can we make people heal? No, we can't. Everyone's walk is unique to them. Some start on the path weeks after loss; for others it's years; for some it may take decades, and for others, unhappily, it never happens.

When my heart started to mend, I knew it would be a very different shape from what it had been before, and that was okay. In fact, that was better, as I wanted loss to have changed me. My heart was now bigger than ever, because the love for my children had expanded its capacity, so a new shape was a good thing.

Are there obstacles that can make healing harder for some people? Yes, there are:

Personality: How we journey through loss and life in general can be shaped by our personality and character traits.

Upbringing: How we are raised, and the skills we have developed through life experiences, definitely play a part in how we recover from trauma and loss.

Lack of joy: If a person's life has no hope within it, or they have nothing to look forward to in the future, recovery from trauma and loss is more challenging.

To recap:
- I was broken
- My heart was rebuilt in a different shape from before
- I am no longer broken, my heart did heal, but I am forever changed

How I started on the path to healing my heart:

- I kept talking about the loss and my experiences – talking is key to the brain and heart accepting what has happened, and it helps any trauma connected to the loss(es) to be processed.

- I gave myself permission to visit the pain whenever I felt it was needed – I didn't run from it or deny it was there; I was willing to face it head-on.

- I spoke about the loss – I refused to let it become a taboo, and that meant I could process the grief, and other people then felt equally comfortable talking about loss around me.

- I stopped trying to recover and to move through grief faster. You simply can't rush grief and the more you try, the slower you journey through it. If you can lay down all your expectations and just go at your own pace, grieving becomes a much easier process.

- I stopped trying to be happy again. I decided that to be happy in the immediate aftermath was out of my reach, so I decided to just live to make others happy. By doing this I unexpectedly rediscovered my smile and joy.

- I re-engaged with life. By joining in things with your family, friends and community you see that life can bring you happy moments again, and, while this is hard to accept at first, it makes life more tolerable moving forwards.

- I started to look after myself again. In the initial part of the grieving process I stopped caring about what I looked like; in fact, the worse I looked, the better I felt, as I felt the outside then showed a glimmer of what I was feeling like on the inside. After some time, I decided to start taking care of myself again, and, while it felt like an effort initially, it made me feel more like me again and that helped in the long run.

- I engaged with others who had experienced similar loss, and hearing that many of my experiences were shared by them helped me feel less alone.

This is my walk.

This is my path.

Your path will be unique to you.

How you heal is personal to you, and nothing is wrong and nothing is right in the way you journey your way through grief.

Please can I encourage you to be fearless in addressing the pain you are experiencing; don't run from the grief, face it head-on.

We cannot ever judge another grieving person, or critique how they heal, or don't heal; all we can do is cheer them on and help them on their walk. I hope explaining how I have healed helps you in some way.

Losing a person you love in no way means you are automatically doomed to be sad forever – this is what I needed to hear, and so I wanted to tell you.

THE QUEST FOR HAPPINESS

I spent endless nights wailing on the floor, repeating over and over, 'I just want to be happy again – someone tell me how to be happy.' Losing my sense of happiness was probably a major layer of my grief pie. I had always considered myself a truly happy, joy-filled person, and to have this part of me suddenly remove felt like I lost my identity. I didn't recognise this sad, heartbroken person staring back at me in the mirror. The eyes that used to shine with expectation and excitement now looked lifeless and terrified – who was I without a smile on my face?

I guess this is when my quest to discover what happiness truly meant began. Maybe true happiness could still be found following heartbreak and loss; maybe, just maybe, I could still be happy, even in the depths of grief – perhaps one can be in mourning and still be a happy person?

So, what did this quest look like in practical terms? I started by acknowledging all the beautiful things I still had in my life. I won't bore you with listing them here, as your list would be unique to you and comparison helps no one. But we all have something to be grateful for. Perhaps it is your partner, your soulmate; maybe it's having lots of friends to support you, or one special friend who has been able to carry you through tragedy – whatever or whoever you include on your list, just by taking time to consider how blessed you are to have them in your life can tweak your perspective on life, and it definitely changed mine.

I chose not to say, 'Why me?' Instead I said, 'Why not me?' This stopped me feeling victimised by life, and made me face the fact that these terrible things happen to many people (too many people), and I wasn't being singled out. It wasn't because I deserved it, or that life was picking on me – it's simply the nature of loss and grief; it doesn't discriminate, it targets anyone and everyone.

I decided to let go of the deep desperation to feel happy again – the more I talked about the loss of my joy and the more I dissected why I couldn't be happy again, the sadder I felt.

I had to choose to let it go, and say if I am never happy again, then that is okay. Is it what I desired? No. Would I like it to be different? Yes. But longing for it doesn't bring it back.

Next, I decided to read about people who had overcome tragedy. I soaked up every story I could find about those who had been broken by life, but had somehow continued on. This stopped me feeling sorry for myself and made me look in awe at these amazing people who are dotted around the globe. People who you would think should be rocking in a corner, but who are instead leading meaningful lives. I saw how loss had transformed their souls – and I made a choice to be one of these people. That didn't mean I needed to do something extraordinary, or build the world's biggest orphanage, it just meant I wasn't going to let loss destroy my future; I was going to find hope in the darkness. I noticed that none of these beautiful humans talked much about happiness – as happiness was a small emotion compared to what they were feeling and expressing.

Anything can make you happy, and happiness is a transient state and emotion. Being fulfilled, hope-filled, compassionate, empathetic and a good human are all way more important.

I said to Andy that we needed to do something for people who are desperate and unhappy right now. It didn't matter what it was, but I needed to know that what we did would help someone feel cared for. We chose to make hampers for people who were alone and lonely, massive hampers that would feed them for weeks. It was a big task and took us weeks to do – but boy did it feel good to know people wouldn't be going hungry, and also would feel loved.

Then we put together rucksacks for people who were homeless – these included sleeping bags, socks, wet wipes, mints, notepad and pens, tissues, toothbrushes and so much more. We then handed them to groups working with homeless people across two cities. Again, this took us weeks – but we felt like we were doing something to help other people and I can't tell you how good that felt. It didn't matter that we were sobbing while putting these packs together; we did it anyway, and we knew our pain was being ploughed into helping other people.

These are just two of the many things we did, and I can wholeheartedly recommend you do something that removes you from your own pain for a short amount of time, and makes you look at the wider world.

(My only word of caution here is: don't volunteer for things and not follow through; charities have so few resources and when people let them down it really affects them. Also, don't offer to do anything that means you need to provide emotional support – wait until your heart has mended to do that.)

A massive milestone then happened: I gave myself permission to feel joy again. Me smiling didn't mean I didn't love the ones I had lost, and it didn't mean I wasn't hurting anymore. So I watched as much stand-up comedy as I could. I watched Nigella cooking delicious food, Oprah conducting inspiring interviews and *The Vicar of Dibley* on repeat on TV. If it was going to make me laugh or smile, or bring me any enjoyment, I said, 'Yes, please, bring it on.'

I then wrote down how I was feeling, on notepads, in journals, anywhere I could find space to express my feelings. Pain needs a voice at times, and if we can let it flow out of us in words, it can help the brain accept the circumstances we now live in.

I explored my faith more. Some find faith through loss, some reject it, and others go deeper into it. I was already a committed Christian, and I have to say that having a faith really did help me, way more than I could say in just one paragraph.

I think loss often makes people look into the meaning of life, or other deep life issues, and I completely understand why, as you just feel so small and insignificant. My faith helped me as it made me look beyond this world, and while this world seemed full of pain that was a much-needed respite.

Next, I stopped delaying my happiness with thoughts such as: 'If x happens, I will feel happy again. If y and z happen, I will find my peace.' It was time to stop postponing things and making excuses for why I couldn't feel it. I could feel happy right now if I chose to – even in the depths of my darkness. I could be a happy person and a broken person.

Over time, it then happened. Not in a way I imagined it to happen. I wanted to be as happy as I was prior to going through loss and grief, and to my surprise I was now happier than I had been before.

Life had more meaning. The depth of pain I had experienced created new, much deeper reserves in my soul (and, yes, it scared me that a human could feel that much sorrow), but post-loss those reserves could be filled with joy, and as they were now way deeper they could hold so much more happiness.

I can't promise you this is a foolproof way to rediscover happiness; all I can say is this is how I found mine again. If any of this helps lead you to the path to find your smile, I will be delighted.

If you ask me who I like to spend time with, I would tell you this. Let me sit amongst those who have known suffering, those who have been to hell and back, when they waded through the valley of despair. They are the ones who wear their heart on their sleeve. They often hate polite chit-chat, as they know life is far too short for superficial conversation. They speak about issues that truly matter, and they connect with others deeply. They value relationship, and when they make a friend, it is a friend for life. Why? Well pain reveals people and it shines a light on things of true significance. My advice to anyone is to search out these precious souls, and make them your best friends. They will make your life richer simply by being in it.

ZOË CLARK-COATES

10 QUESTIONS

I am always amazed at the diverse questions that I get asked at events and on social media, and I thought it might be helpful to include some of my favourites here as they may give you an insight into my thinking and stance on life.

1. What shocked you about grief?

Many, many things. I may have trained as a counsellor prior to experiencing loss, but nothing in the world could have prepared me for walking the path I did.

~ One thing that surprised me was that my heart wasn't just broken because of the losses; my heart also broke due to the mammoth disappointment I was carrying, and due to the terror of the unknown. The agony was kind of surreal, and it made me feel like I had left the planet and had transcended to a different universe.

~ I was shocked at the million questions that rushed around my brain. The: 'What if you don't survive this?' 'What if you are broken forever?' 'What if you never stop crying?' Oh, the questions, the never-ending questions of a brain that seems to seek to destroy you when you are deeply broken.

I found the only way to survive this was not to torture myself with seeking the answers; I simply kept telling myself the same thing on repeat: 'Then I will survive it.' I gave in to the pain, I submitted to the questions that only grief born from deep love can pose and, over time, the questions stopped – but nothing could have prepared me for this part of grief.

~ I was so shocked at the immense fear I experienced. Grief really does throw you into a huge black pit. C. S. Lewis said, 'nothing prepared me for the fact that grief looks so like fear'. And boy does that quote ring true.

Grief does look so like terror; it is daunting and all-consuming. I feared everything. I feared waking up each morning as I knew I would have to live through another day of fresh pain. I feared going to sleep because of the nightmares. Often when you have a bad dream you wake up and reassure yourself that it is just a dream and nothing to be scared of, but during that time I would wake up and realise the nightmare was real, it was true life – that really terrified me.

- The most shocking thing was that the blackest grief, the haunting, harrowing, please-kill-me-now type of grief, did end. For a long time I didn't think it would, but it did. It gradually changed and became less and less. I would no longer say I am mourning. While I am fully aware grief is a lifelong passage, I don't feel broken any longer. In fact, I feel more whole than I have ever been, and happier than ever – I never believed that was possible in the aftermath of loss.

- One thing I have noticed when walking with the dying and the bereaved is that grief can make people lose their filter, and this can be both beautiful and incredibly painful. You might get to hear heartfelt truths, or they might recount stories that have never previously been shared; but they can also say things that aren't always kind, or well thought through, so you have to constantly remind yourself to respond with grace.

2. What was the worst part of loss for you?

I think one of the worst parts was feeling like the pain was infinite. There was no end in sight, and that is a truly hard thing to live with. The most harrowing part of loss was knowing that however long I waited and however many tears I wept, my loved ones were never coming back.

Over time I was able to accept that, while their physical

presence here with me was limited, the love I carried for them was never-ending, and that meant they will always be part of me, and that helped ease the pain.

3. Where did you find strength?

My strength came when I said I will no longer run from this pain. I faced the battle; with shaking legs and a quivering lip, I said I will not hide from the agony, I will process it. Even if that meant wailing on the floor in a pool of tears.

To be expected to face another day on this planet while carrying the weight of grief on your shoulders is similar to being asked to reside in a lion's cage. Daunting, terrifying and incomprehensible. And to need to find any kind of strength when you feel broken is pretty impossible, so I tell everyone not to even look for it. Your only task is to take one step forwards today; you don't need to find any hidden reserve – strength will find you, if you don't find it. Whether it finds you in that pool of tears in the valley, or while you are walking on a mountain top – wherever you may be, it will sneak up on you, I promise you.

I also want to say that while I was waiting for strength to find me, I found me!

4. How did you feel ready to move on with life?

If I always waited until I felt mentally or emotionally ready for things, I promise you I would do nothing. My secret? I show up, however I feel.

I also decided very early on that I would never ask, 'Why is this happening to me?' I always thought, 'Why shouldn't this be happening to me.'

This stopped me feeling like a victim of circumstance. I also decided to learn from everything – to constantly look for a hidden lesson, or a gift or a blessing, even in the deepest of traumas (which, believe me, isn't easy). I can hand-on-heart say this was a big game-changer for me, as it made me look more positively at things.

5. What do you wish someone had told you when you were going through grief?

- Grief can make you hide in the shadows, but it helps to lean into the light. I was so scared to show the real me, the broken me, and it often felt easier to hide that pain away. But if we courageously choose to be vulnerable and let the light hit our faces, we can crawl through the valley of darkness much more easily. Often, we find others who are also crawling, and these people can become lifelong friends – I call them 'valley friends'. They have walked the same path, or perhaps dragged themselves along the same path, and they are usually the people who understand you the most.

- The pain is not limited, as the love is endless. Knowing this would have helped me understand and accept the pain I was going through.

- You don't need to fight to survive. I often used to scream that I couldn't make it through another day, and I didn't want to live a moment longer with the raw agony that only loss can bring. After some time, I discovered I didn't need to fight the pain; the only thing I needed to do was open my eyes when I woke up and bravely look at the heartbreak and refuse to run from it. To have been told this would have helped me a lot.

- There will be days when you are hit by a fresh wave of grief and you will doubt how far you have swum in the ocean of mourning. Let me reassure you that these waves are part of the journey, they won't put you back. In fact, they do the exact opposite; they carry you forwards if you don't fight them – just hold onto your life ring and let the current carry you on.

You won't drown and you may need to tell yourself this a hundred times a day. Let it become your mantra: 'I won't drown; I am just learning to swim.'

- When walking through grief, feelings change by the hour – heck, let's be even more realistic, they change by the second. So, if someone asks you if you are okay now, that doesn't mean you need to be okay in 60 minutes, or that you were okay yesterday. Just try to stay as present as you can.

- Grief isn't something you can control. I think a huge misconception about grief is that it is controllable, that people can choose when and where to feel it and process it, and before going through loss I probably believed this a little too, if I'm honest. Once you have experienced grief first-hand you can only laugh at this myth. Can you control love? No, of course you can't; love is a powerful force that controls people, and the same applies to grief, and we must respect that. Knowing this would have helped me no end.

◈ Sometimes all the explaining in the world won't help others understand loss and grief. People will always view things from their own level of perception and from their own personal experience.

6. Did grief bring you any gifts?

◈ Grief made me rip up the rule book. Suddenly I got to just be me. I stopped wanting to conform and please those around me. Maybe I was beyond caring? Perhaps I was so broken I felt no shame in sobbing on the floor? Whatever the case, it brought me a freedom to be truly authentic and that really is a gift.

◈ My loved ones were robbed of all their tomorrows, but because of them I embrace all of my todays – that is a gift.

◈ It's in the brokenness . . .
It's in the waiting . . .
It's in the pain . . .
It's in the darkest of places . . .
that we discover the depth of the love we are able to feel. That is a gift.

7. Why does grief make people feel out of control?

We all like to control our destiny and there is nothing more out of our control than grief. It's not possible for us to predict or defer death, and as such we can't stop grief from entering our lives. Grief brings with it chaos. It collects every element of our lives, puts it all into a big basket and then shakes it.

Things may break in that basket, things will certainly change shape, and the pieces will always come out in a strange and confusing order. No part of this is easy to bear.

Many assume grief needs to be conquered, but, actually, it is something people need to face and not fight. This takes a real leap of faith and a complete release of control. It takes real trust to let it surround you like fog on a mountain top, but eventually a path will open up before you and you can step straight through it.

8. What would you say to someone who is trying to stop a family member or friend from crying?

☞ When you see someone crying, please remember tears have a voice. That voice is so rarely listened to; it is mostly ignored and told to stay quiet for fear of inducing more weeping. But something magical happens if we listen. Those droplets of water speak the profound truth, and tell life-changing stories – so listen to those teardrops.

☞ To have someone catch every tear is a beautiful gift – you can give that gift to a bereaved person.

☞ It's easy to sit on the shoreline and judge those swimming in the ocean of grief, but unless you have nearly drowned at sea, say nothing more than 'Can I send help to you?' or 'How can I help you?' – never 'Perhaps you should stop crying'.

I think the world can wrongly think it helps others to try to look for a bright side even in tragedy. But sometimes there isn't a bright side, however much people want there to be. Sometimes it's just crap. Agonisingly painful. Overwhelmingly terrible – and we just have to accept that, and give people the freedom to sob.

Sometimes people just need to be lifted onto another's shoulders so they can see over the parapet of grief. Your shoulders may be good for that.

Remember, grief is sacred; it is liquid love streaming from the cracks of a broken heart. Please don't fear it.

9. What do you want people to know about people who are grieving?

Bereaved people frequently feel pressured not to talk of the person they have lost, because society wants to avoid mentioning them by name. It's as if the bereaved are being forced to rip out the pages of their life story where their loved ones reside. But the bereaved usually want their loved ones to be celebrated. You can help this happen by talking about these precious people and by not fearing the subject of loss.

Be aware that it is pretty hard to articulate the pain. Most people are taught the language to express joy, but there are rarely lessons in how to communicate devastating loss.

I had no clue how to express that my world was unravelling in front of my eyes, and most people are the same.

Give people time and space to find the words they need to convey their experience. Sometimes they may be so numb and overwhelmed with grief that the only thing they are able to do is sit and stare at a wall. In those moments, all they need is for you to sit and stare at the wall with them.

- People crave normality and often want to do normal everyday things without fear of judgement.

- If everyone surrounding those bereaved recognises the loss, it means the individual/couple can focus on grieving, rather than utilising their small reserves of energy to defend their right to grieve.

- That when a person dies it is not only a story of pain; there is also beauty in the ashes.

10. What words would you whisper into a bereaved person's ear today?

Maybe today you are looking at people on Instagram or Facebook, or at others in your life, and thinking, 'How? How on earth have they got to the stage in life where they are happy? How have they run the race and are still here to tell the tale?' Well, let me reassure you of this:

I had no clue how I was going to get to the finish line. I didn't even know how I was going to get over the starting line, but I just kept stepping forwards and, before I knew it, I was on my way. So, I am here to cheer you on and be that small voice you need to hear telling you, 'You can do this and you will survive.'

QUESTIONS I ASKED THE BEREAVED

Can you tell me what you wish you had known at the start of your journey through loss?

- How utterly alone I would feel, as it scared me to feel this so powerfully.

- That it's okay to feel the way I felt, as society made me feel like a freak for feeling the way I did.

- That there is a taboo surrounding the subject of death, as I couldn't understand why people shut down the moment I opened up about my pain.

- To get help when needed, as I felt ashamed to reach out for support. I also felt the loss was my fault, and of course it wasn't.

- I wish I had known that grief can cause both physical and emotional pain. The physical pain affected my whole body and I was simply unprepared for that.

- I wish I'd known that the raw pain and shock doesn't last forever.

- That it's okay to cry – no, more than that, that it's healthy to cry, as I spent a lot of time trying to put a brave face on for the world.

- I wish I had known that many people would not understand my grief as they hadn't personally encountered a loss like mine. So many people had very little empathy, compassion or understanding of what I was going through. I would have loved for someone to have told me that this lack of empathy from others didn't mean my grief was invalid. No one should have to justify grieving for anyone. I would now say, surround yourself with those who are compassionate and distance yourself when possible from those who aren't, just like Zoë said in her book *Saying Goodbye*. Removing yourself from people who simply don't get it does not make you a bad person; it means you just have self-respect and want others to be compassionate about your pain and journey.

- I wish I had known I would survive, because I didn't think I would. I couldn't see life being anything other than grief-filled. Going through loss changed me in more ways than I thought possible, but it doesn't define me anymore.

- I wish somebody had warned me of what grief really felt like and that I wasn't going crazy. The emotional impact, feeling like I was the only one in the world and thinking that I was going mad, led to self-hatred.

What was the most helpful thing anyone said to you about loss and grief?

- The words 'it's okay to feel the way you feel, it's okay to cry and you must take time to grieve', were a godsend, as they gave me permission to embrace the grieving process. I also needed people to reassure me that it was not my fault, but to validate my feelings, as I felt angry, guilty, anxious and sad, all at the same time.

- It was something you said actually, Zoë, and it was this: That I was grieving as much as I was, because I loved them as much as I did; this gave me a sense of gratitude for the grief I was feeling, and stopped me resenting it as much.

- To not feel shame or weak when grieving. I think the world tells us strength is putting a brave face on, but actually true courage is being real about the feelings we are encountering.

- The most helpful thing I heard during that time was that grief affects everyone in different ways, as that made me feel okay with the fact that I wasn't experiencing similar things to others in my family.

- That grief isn't neatly packaged. It's messy and often feels like a bomb has been detonated in your life.

- That it's okay not to be okay; to process it as quickly or as slowly as I wished, and not to be afraid to ask for help when it is needed.

- Eat crap, watch crap, stay in bed, anything goes – just don't get drunk alone.

- Your partner may well grieve in a different way and/or at a different time – this can be hard but it is okay. There is no standard pattern of grief. Some days one of you may feel nothing. Some days you feel everything. Accepting that is so important.

- Hearing grief described as a spiral by Zoë in one of her books was so helpful to me, as it is so apt and I wish I had heard this immediately after loss. Sometimes all the emotions came back at unexpected moments and it felt like I was right back in that place when it happened, when time stopped. But I wasn't like that even though it felt like I was; I was one step further on.

- The most helpful thing was 'I'm so sorry for your loss' and just crying with me or sitting with me while I cried.

How do you feel you have changed post-loss?

- I don't think I'm quite as optimistic as I once was. But I am on a journey to rebuild the life that was given to me.

- I would always overthink situations and worry about people's perceptions of me. I have a new-found inner confidence and belief in myself. I have empathy for strangers and a natural desire to help others. I don't worry about what others think, I am content in the life I lead.

- I never thought I would say this but as a person I believe I am now happier – our journey has been tough; at times I have been bitter, angry, resentful, lost friends and hidden away from the world. However, I have also made friends for life post-loss, people whose path I may never have crossed had we not lost our son.

- I feel I am able to express my feelings more openly to my family and friends. I also strongly believe that I appreciate life way more post-loss. I suppose it's given me a different perspective on life. I always knew the time on earth we have is limited, but losing someone you love makes you understand that at a deeper level.

- I feel more grateful for things; I take nothing for granted anymore.

- I am much more able to feel empathy for others in the same position and feel better placed to support people through loss and grief because of my experience.

- I count my blessings more and try to focus on the here and now, rather than worrying about the future.

- I'm kinder to myself and feel more in touch with my emotions than I have ever been. There are times when I'm more guarded than I once was, though, as I am nervous of encountering more pain.

- I am more compassionate, empathetic, understanding and gracious. I have a different perspective on life, valuing people, family and love above all else. My marriage is stronger because of the grief we have journeyed together. My mental health is stronger as I have had to work so hard at dealing with my trauma.

- I have felt pain with every fibre of my being; it has consumed and engulfed me at times, but I also love with an intensity I didn't have before. Grief has given me the gift to overcome. To really see the pain in the world and not shy away from it. To feel it, but not dwell in hopelessness.

Following deep loss people can be scared of feeling happy again. You see sadness and heartbreak have resided for so long, even the thought of feeling joy makes them feel disloyal to the grief. So how does one help? You show understanding, empathy and reassure them that the power of their love transcends everything. As you pour on them grace and kindness, they will (in time) discover this new world they reside in can hold both pain and joy simultaneously, and whether they are weeping or smiling their loved one will forever be honoured.

ZOË CLARK-COATES

PART 2

60 Days of Support
and Journalling

DAY 1

Wanting to hide away following mind-blowing grief is not just expected, it is totally normal. It doesn't mean you are having a breakdown, or have suddenly developed a panic disorder; it simply means you need time out, and time to process what you have just experienced. So be gentle with yourself. Allow the tears to fall, eat chocolate, eat comforting soup, do whatever you need to do to survive in the aftermath.

TASK FOR THE DAY

Write here how you feel. Be honest. Be raw. This is your space to process your feelings.

It's understandable that you choose to
hide under your duvet.

It is totally fine to slip down a wall, screaming
and shouting that life isn't fair.

It is okay that you stand in the shower with
tears streaming down your face faster than the
jets of water spraying your body.

Grief hurts.

Loss is mind-blowing.

Heartbreak is earth-shattering.

Whatever you need to do to survive is FINE.

ZOË CLARK-COATES

DAY 2

Self-care. It is normal not to want to look after yourself following loss, but I urge you to ignore the desire to forget you, because *you* matter. Often people see little purpose in eating well, or trying to rest, and not doing these things can almost feel like an act of self-expression, as you are showing the world that life is too hard and you want to give up. But it is essential that you do look after yourself, so you can regain your strength.

TASK FOR THE DAY

- Shower.
- Find your most favourite item of clothing and wear it.
- What do you love to eat? Cook it or buy it.
- What is your favourite movie? Watch it.
- What is your favourite book? Dig it out and reread it.
- Where is your favourite walk? Can you go there and breathe in fresh air?
- Who is your favourite person to chat with? Call them.
- Today is about you. Today is about acknowledging you matter.

Our lost loved one is not pain, they are not a wound, they are not the trauma – the loss is the agony, not the precious soul that was taken from us far too soon. So, when people say, 'Maybe you are best not to talk about them in case you reopen the wound' or 'Perhaps you are making it worse', they are simply not understanding that they were a gift. They are the beautiful treasure people spend their life searching for. By talking about them, we heal. By sharing their story, however short or long it may have been, we cast a light in someone else's dark world. And, perhaps most importantly, we are acknowledging they were here, that their lives made a difference, that because they existed we are different – that, because of them, the world is a better place.

ZOË CLARK-COATES

DAY 3

I think many of us are taught to put pain into a nice neat parcel and hide it away, as we are encouraged by society to just put on a brave face and get on with life. While we do need to carry on with life – as sadly our bills still need to be paid, so we can keep a roof over our heads – we definitely should not be encouraged to run from pain. Sometimes we just need to yield to the agony, and immerse ourselves in our feelings and emotions so we can process them. Once they are processed and our brain has reluctantly come to terms with the trauma we have faced, the healing can commence.

TASK FOR THE DAY

What do you feel society is saying to you? Write down five messages you are hearing from those around you. Now consider if these are helpful. If they aren't helpful, consider how you should respond and move forwards.

1 _____

2 _____

3 _____

4 _____

5 _____

The day after I heard of their death, what shocked me the most was that the sun still rose, and the post still slipped through my mailbox, and I still got thirsty, and the birds still sang, and the traffic lights still changed colour . . . but my world had stopped, my planet had stopped spinning.

ZOË CLARK-COATES

DAY 4

We all have dreams and we all have a vision of how our life should look. Loss doesn't take these hopes and plans into account, it just rips them up in front of our eyes. I think one of the key parts of grief is accepting that in the briefest of moments life changed forever, that it no longer resembles what we had planned. This means processing the shock. Accepting the painful reality of life now being different, and then being willing to consider a new plan and a different future. None of this is easy, it is incredibly difficult, but once we have considered a new way forwards it makes life feel a little more stable and back in control.

TASK FOR THE DAY

What three things would help you move forwards? Do you need to see a doctor and talk about your physical/emotional health? Do you need to change things at work? Do you need to join an exercise programme, so you feel fitter and stronger? Do you need to spend less time on social media, and more time enjoying nature?

1 _____

2 _____

3 _____

The mistake so many make when trying to help the bereaved is they tell those in mourning they should be thankful for having a heart that still beats in their chest. It is as though they feel that reminding them they have so much more life to live will encourage them to re-find their purpose. The truth is, this will never bring comfort to the broken-hearted; they feel no gratitude in being alive, they are just being made to feel guilty for wanting to die. So, if you want to help the grieving, don't tell them they should feel thankful, don't tell them they 'should' feel anything, just allow them to be, allow them to weep and allow them to crawl through the agony of loss – and, if you want to show love, get on your knees and silently crawl with them.

ZOË CLARK-COATES

DAY 5

Many associate the pain they are feeling with the loss they have experienced, and therefore fear letting go of the pain. They worry that if they don't experience the agony, they won't feel close to the person they have lost. Let me reassure you: your loved one isn't in the pain, they are in the love. The love that will never end. The love that will never dissipate. The love that will never be hidden. The pain can leave, the tears can go, and you will still be forever connected, by your endless, everlasting love.

TASK FOR THE DAY

Find a poem or a song that helps you express the love you feel.

It is okay to love them forever. It is okay to speak of them. It is okay to miss them endlessly. It is okay to be confused. It is okay to be lost and fear never being found. It is okay to be scared of the darkness and long to see the light. It is okay to crave the old you while changing into the new you. It is okay to wish it was different and to dream of a happier ending.

This is the nature of grief, where everything is questioned. When you need reassurance that things are 'okay'. Where you long to be told you aren't going mad, you aren't 'abnormal'.

So let me be the one to tell you this truth . . .

You are normal.

You just loved them more than words can ever say.

Your heart just broke into so many pieces that breathing alone is an effort.

Hold onto this knowledge . . . Grief is a fast-moving river, and as you grieve you are moving downstream.

Let the current take you; you don't need to cling to the river bank.

Even though you don't know how to swim, I promise you this . . .

You will be okay.

ZOË CLARK-COATES

DAY 6

Friends can be such a great support when you are going through loss. Of course, there can be the odd person who isn't the greatest at emotional support, but there are also often unexpected treasures, people you never thought would show up in your moment of need who blow you away with their kindness. I always say grief is the ultimate life sieve – it reveals what matters and shows you people's true characters. While this sieve can unearth some potential issues, it can also make life so much richer for you in the future, so try to embrace it and not fear it.

TASK FOR THE DAY

Which of your friends have been your lifeline? Have any of your friends surprised you with their kindness and love?

Write down three things that have been true gifts to you, so you never forget them.

1 _____

2 _____

3 _____

They were here,
then they were gone.
The care (or the lack of care),
the support (or the lack of support),
the kindness (or the lack of kindness)
during that time stays with you forever.

ZOË CLARK-COATES

DAY 7

So many people worry that they shouldn't talk of the person they have lost. They fear others may think they aren't coping, or are dwelling in misery, or perhaps even seeking attention. Oh, how untrue these things are. Talking of the person you have lost does nothing more than show the world you have lost the one you adore. I know I say a lot throughout this book that talking is key, but that's only because it is so true, and people don't need to hear this only once, they need to hear it over and over again, so they feel encouraged to do it. So, let me encourage you to keep talking about your feelings, keep talking about the pain, so your heart and brain can start to heal.

TASK FOR THE DAY

Write down what you want the world to know about the person you have loved and lost.

People need to be reminded that they can survive the passage of grief. It is so easy to forget that when fumbling around in the darkness of the pit. So let me be the one to remind you today. You will make it through. You will rediscover your joy. You will flourish again, and you will do it to honour the one you have lost.

ZOË CLARK-COATES

DAY 8

How do you accept something that feels so utterly wrong? It is easy to accept things that have gone right, but how does something painful or crippling ever sit comfortably in your soul? I don't think it can, to be honest. Some things will never make sense, and will never, ever be okay – and that is what we have to come to terms with. It is only when life (or people) force us to try to be okay with what has happened that this internal fight occurs; the peace can only come when we accept that it doesn't make sense. That it is completely wrong. That how we envisioned life to look has been shattered, and we never need to be okay with that; we can just move forwards accepting that life is sometimes crap.

TASK FOR THE DAY

Take time out from thinking today, whether that be 15 minutes or 5 minutes. Free your mind from questions and expectations. Lie down, put on some music and just be. If thoughts pop into your mind, don't engage with them. Just focus on the music and let the bed or floor absorb your weight. This is your time to escape and give your brain a chance to rest.

Small things can trigger a fresh wave of grief – a smell, a look or perhaps a song – and within seconds you are flung into a time machine and are transported back to that 'moment' when time stood still, and the world had crashed at your feet.

ZOË CLARK-COATES

DAY 9

~~~~~~

When you lose a person you love you aren't just losing them at the age at which they died – you are losing them at every age they have yet to celebrate. This is why grief is a lifelong journey, as you will always be acutely aware of how old your loved one should be at every point in your life. While this can seem daunting early on in the grief journey, to even contemplate the walk of grief being so long, I can assure you it won't always feel like that. Once the acute pain subsides and the blackest part of grief fades, you just journey on with this awareness and it becomes part of who you are. People often assume grief is just about pain, but it isn't; it is also about expressing and carrying love.

TASK FOR THE DAY

What three things are you most sad about not knowing or seeing? For me, I wish I could have known what my children's personalities would have been like and what hobbies they would have enjoyed. Perhaps you are sad that your dad won't now get to walk you down the aisle? Or that your mum won't get to hold her first grandchild. Perhaps you are grieving for that holiday you had always talked about with your partner and never took? This is your space to openly consider your feelings.

1 _____

2 _____

3 _____

~ ~

When you survive loss, everyone is quick to tell
you how strong you are and how tough you must be.
But actually, no one has a choice to survive grief, do they?
It's not optional. You just have to cry in the shower,
sob into your pillow and pray you will make it.

~ ~ ~ ~ ~ ~ ~ ~ ~ ~ ZOË CLARK-COATES ~ ~ ~ ~ ~ ~ ~ ~ ~ ~ ~

DAY 10

When I hear people say they are fighting back the tears, my first question is always: why? Why would you want to fight away this beautiful expression of emotion? Tears have a voice, and that voice is so rarely listened to, but something magical happens if we do listen to what the tears are saying. Those droplets of water speak profound truth and tell life-changing stories. So, let me encourage you to weep whenever you need to. Sob on the floor. Howl in the shower. Fill your pillow with tears. Let your tears tell your story, and they will transport you to a place of healing.

TASK FOR THE DAY

Go to a private place where you fear no judgement and let the tears flow. Don't let that inner voice tell you not to go there in case you can't stop once you have started; this will just keep you locked in the pain. Cry. Release the pain, which will in turn release the hormones and chemicals which tears of grief contain. Expect to feel drained following a release of powerful emotion, so ensure you have the time to recompose yourself, or a time to rest or even sleep.

I often used to say, 'I am fine, thank you' when people asked me how I was. Their response would just be to say, 'Great', and on we all moved. What I longed for them to say was, 'I know you aren't fine, but one day you will be.' To simply know my pain was acknowledged and my aching heart was being heard would have meant the world. This is the gift we can all give to anyone who is walking the path of grief. Listen to their whispers and breathe life into aching souls.

ZOË CLARK-COATES

DAY 11

I don't know if you are like me, but I fear looking weak, and worry that people may think I am not coping. I think it is odd that these worries ever even enter our mind, and maybe that's a society issue? Or perhaps it's due to how we were raised, if we have been conditioned to think of others before we consider what is actually best for our own well-being? Whatever the reason, there comes a time when we need to forget what others think, and be true to ourselves. When we fight conformity and embrace true self-expression, amazing things can happen – not only can we begin to heal, we also give others the freedom to be true to themselves.

TASK FOR THE DAY

Do you feel you act in a certain way due to societal pressure or because those around you have told you to conform? Do you feel you would be happier and more at peace if you acted differently from these expectations? If the answer is yes, consider how you can make changes. Going through significant loss blows your world to pieces, and at times you can make real changes as your life starts to be rebuilt. You don't need to put all the pieces back into the same place!

People told me I was brave not to give up,
but want to know the truth? I did give up! We all give
up! When the pain is all-consuming, when life has lost
all meaning, we all scream at the sky, 'Enough!' But
something magical happens when we quit; when we
say, 'I can't take any more!' We discover life carries on
regardless and, when we have nothing more to offer,
a new strength is sent to carry us through.

ZOË CLARK-COATES

DAY 12

People often ask me when the missing them will end. The answer is simple: never! Sometimes this makes me feel like the bearer of bad news, but it is actually a gift. Why would anyone want the missing them to end? If you didn't miss them, it would mean you were glad they had left, and of course you would never feel like that. So why is missing them a gift? Well, for me, the missing them shows the world and myself that I loved them endlessly. It shows that they left a space in my life that can never and should never be filled by anyone, as only they can fit that exact space. It also shows one other important thing – it shows that they mattered then, they matter now and they will always matter.

TASK FOR THE DAY

Try to rewire your thinking. The world tells us that missing people is wrong, and we need to move on and get over it. It tells us that missing someone is a curse rather than a blessing. While we feel a need to fight our natural feelings (which are to miss someone forever), we resent having these feelings present in our life, and this can become a source of conflict in our minds. If we can change our thinking and accept it's a gift and a blessing to miss someone, we can find room for these feelings in our life, and naturally adjust to them. Once we accept it's normal and right to feel this way, we also leave no room for feelings of shame and guilt. I promise you that if you can untangle what you have been taught and accept this new way of thinking, it will be life-changing.

❦ ❦

I thought I shouldn't reveal my heart until my life was in perfect order. Oh, how wrong I was. Those who want to make the biggest impact in this world need to share from those broken, messy places. Where the sores have yet to heal and the pieces of their broken heart are clearly visible to anyone who goes looking. There is beauty in the chaos and strength buried among the ashes. Those who are brave enough to be authentic and real, in an era where we are taught to fake it until we make it, are really the world-changers in our society.

❦ ❦ ❦ ❦ ❦ ❦ ❦ ❦ ❦ ZOË CLARK-COATES ❦ ❦ ❦ ❦ ❦ ❦ ❦ ❦ ❦

DAY 13

Chaos.

Grief and loss bring chaos. It is like our lives are put into a washing machine and all hell breaks loose when it's whizzing around in circles. Everything in that machine changes shape. Dye leaks out of items and runs into others. Things that should only be handwashed have also been put in there, and are then destroyed. But what also happens is that some things come out better than before. Some items come out clean and fresh. Some items come out a different shape, but that turns out to be a better fit than before. So, while the washing machine is a harrowing experience, it can reap good things too. So why do I share this? Not because I want you to look on the bright side – as there is *no* bright side when it comes to death and loss – but because I want you to know there is hope post-loss, that good things can be born from tragedy, as I needed to hear this when I was in the depths of loss. I needed someone to be a lighthouse in the darkness, to show me life could be better down the line and some of the pain I was experiencing could be turned into purpose. So try not to give up hope – hold on. The washing machine will eventually stop.

TASK FOR THE DAY

Is there anything you would like to be different post-loss? Would you like to change jobs? Would you like to find new friends? Would you like to take up a different hobby? Would you like to look more at the meaning of life? Use the pain from loss to help transform your life into something better.

It's okay to be different.

It's okay to be bruised.

It is okay to show one's scars . . .

I don't know when the world started to tell us
Perfection was beautiful, but it is wrong.

The truth is, vulnerability is breathtaking.

Being authentic is inspiring and walking with our
head held high,

Carrying no shame from our journey,

Is where real beauty can be found.

ZOË CLARK-COATES

DAY 14

What happens if you can't cry? What happens if the tears just won't flow?

Firstly, don't panic. Sometimes the shock of loss prevents tears from being able to come. A lack of tears does not mean you don't love the one you have lost, and it certainly doesn't mean you didn't care. Everyone is different, and for some their natural response may not be to weep on the floor; it may be to write a song, or run a marathon. Grief can be expressed in so many different ways and what I hope you have learnt from this book is that grief is as personal as your fingerprint. So, the only important thing is finding your way to express your grief so that it can be channelled and processed.

TASK FOR THE DAY

Can you think of different ways you can express your grief? Write a list of ways you could express the pain you are feeling, which would help you move through the grieving process.

1 _____

2 _____

3 _____

4 _____

The thing with grief is it can catch you when you least expect it. Maybe that's in a shop where you see an item of clothing that your loved one would have cherished. Maybe it's at the park when you see a new mother pushing along her baby in a sparkling new pram. Perhaps it's when you are lying in bed at night and the pillow next to you is missing your soulmate's dent. Whenever and wherever it catches you, it's gut-wrenching and has the power to leave you speechless.

ZOË CLARK-COATES

DAY 15

Past trauma.

Remember I previously mentioned that grief is the ultimate life sieve? This really comes into effect when a person has been through previous life traumas or upsets, as grief can bring any unresolved pain or issues to the surface. There really couldn't be a worse time to have to deal with these old emotional scars: when you are grieving, the grief alone is utterly overwhelming without having to deal with old life issues as well, but sadly we often have no control over them resurfacing. You have two options if/when this happens: 1. You can find a way to shove these emotions back into the box from which they emerged (which is tricky, but is sometimes possible); 2. You use this time to deal with the unhealed wounds. Yes, the timing is rubbish, but by dealing with them you are giving yourself the best chance possible of a happier life. If you feel flooded and overwhelmed, I would strongly recommend seeking external help from a professional therapist, who can help you untangle the turmoil. Use this time of grieving to heal and resist the urge to put a cork in the bottle and throw it out to sea.

TASK FOR THE DAY

Has grief brought past upset to the surface for you? If it
has, consider how you could/should deal with it. Do you
need professional help? Or do you just need to sit and talk
with a family member or friend? A helpful exercise can be
to write down all the things that have emerged while you
are grieving and see if there is a common thread to them
all.

Grief is sacred; it is liquid love streaming
from the cracks of a broken heart.

ZOË CLARK-COATES

DAY 16

C. S. Lewis said that he never knew grief felt so like fear, and it is so true. I think grief does feel like fear, but I also think that, when grief consumes you, fear also uses the same door and enters our life. Fear of the future. Fear of what may happen next. Fear of feeling out of control. Fear of the unknown. Fear of more loss. Fear of looking weak. Fear of medical intervention. Fear of how people may react around us. The list goes on and on, as there are a million worries many of us will experience. So how do we cope with the fear? Firstly, I think knowing we are not alone in experiencing this paralysing fear helps greatly, as fear can make us feel isolated and like we are the only one in the world feeling it. I also think that knowing it's common for most people to experience this stops people feeling like they are going crazy. We do have to be careful not to give fear too much space in our minds, however, and also not to give in to the fear. For example, the fear may tell you never to go out just in case you end up crying in public. But a good response to this would be to do the exact thing fear is telling you not to do – go out and if you cry, you cry! Fear will want to lock you into a dark and private cell, so refuse to be trapped by it. Let the inner lion within you roar, and, believe me, fear will eventually flee.

TASK FOR THE DAY

What have you become scared of? How can you fight the fear?

1 _____

✐ I can fight it by

┌──┐
│   │
│   │
└──┘

2 _____

✐ I can fight it by

┌──┐
│   │
│   │
└──┘

✐ ✐

There was a time when I was consumed by fear.

The enemy seemed large and terrifying.

Then I started to develop tenacity and resilience,
and that warrior spirit that had become hidden in
me during the battle rose up once again.

This was a life-changing experience,
my 'Wonder Woman' moment.

I discovered I had more faith than fear,
more hope than doubt. And though I felt weak
I was in fact badass.

✐ ✐ ✐ ✐ ✐ ✐ ✐ ✐ ✐ ✐ ZOË CLARK-COATES ✐ ✐ ✐ ✐ ✐ ✐ ✐ ✐ ✐ ✐

DAY 17

When people ask me to explain what loss is like, the first analogy that leaps to my mind is this. Imagine you are holding onto your loved one's hand over a cliff edge. You are using every bit of strength to hold on to them, but then they let go. You watch them plummet to their death. Everything within you screams 'No!' as you watch them falling. You scream that you never let go, you would never, ever have let go, even if you had died in the process. This wasn't your choice; this wasn't something you could control. Loss is torture. It is hard to explain to someone who has never experienced it, but sometimes it's asked of those who have gone through it to explain, so others who haven't can gain insight.

TASK FOR THE DAY

How would you explain loss? Write down how you explain loss to someone. Sometimes verbalising our pain helps.

What can you do if you don't want to live without someone who has gone? How do you simply survive the pain, the heartbreak, and find your will to continue? Well, you admit how you are feeling. You scream, you shout, you weep on your bedroom floor and you hold on to the edge of that mountain cliff, until your desire to live outweighs your hope to die.

ZOË CLARK-COATES

DAY 18

I love the spring. It feels like it's the start of warmer days and longer evenings . . . however, I didn't always feel like this. There was a period of time where every month was bleak. Seasons blended into one another, and the forecast was always terrifying. So how did this change? Well, it certainly didn't happen overnight! But one day I could see a shoot of new life pushing through the ground, and eventually that turned into the tiniest of flowers. New life and brighter outlooks don't happen as quickly as we may like. Seeds have to be sown and the ground needs to be ready – but then, without any warning, growth starts to happen. The ground starts to move and one tiny bud springs forth. This is enough to give us hope that tomorrow may be brighter, and that life may be worth embracing after all.

TASK FOR THE DAY

Write down what gives you hope that tomorrow may be brighter. What brings you joy, what can bring a smile to your face in the darkest of days?

Initially, the pain was all-consuming. It was like the raw agony had sucked every bit of breath from my lungs. But after some time, the intensity subsided. Was that because the grief was reducing or was it simply because I had become accustomed to living with the weight of the loss? Who knows! But being able to take those shallow breaths again gave me enough oxygen to sustain me to the next day.

ZOË CLARK-COATES

DAY 19

How can a person feel this much pain? A question I would often ask myself, especially in the dark hours of the night when I felt scared due to the volume of pain I was experiencing. The pain felt like a giant before me, and the thought of continuing forwards with this pain hovering over me was beyond daunting. I simply didn't understand how the pain could be so great and so consuming, and then I had a lightbulb moment – the pain was this huge and unending because the love I felt for them was unlimited. With unlimited love comes unlimited pain if the person is lost. This realisation stopped me questioning it, and I accepted it for what it was, and when I stopped fighting the pain, it became less scary. It stopped being an enemy and became an often-silent companion, until it was time for it to leave my life and only the love remained.

TASK FOR THE DAY

Try to write a poem or quote about the pain you are feeling. If you allow yourself to express your pain creatively, it can help transform it.

We all have a view of what 'broken' looks like,
and I think because of this we can assume people who
are broken-hearted are fine if they are smiling.

Please know that grief-stricken people still smile,
they still chat, still engage, still work, still party,
still talk . . . because they have to.

ZOË CLARK-COATES

DAY 20

Can we prepare for loss? No, I don't think we can. We can certainly start grieving before the loss happens, but that is very different from actually preparing for the trap door to open, just in case it does open. If we try to prepare, we just rob ourselves of experiencing true joy in the moment. So often people say to me, 'If only I hadn't made as many plans then it wouldn't hurt as much now.' While it is natural to feel like this, it is not accurate, as the pain of loss is just as huge whether you had plans or not; but one way you experienced the happiness and excitement of dreaming of future events, and the other way you just felt the pain and grief. Your brain may try to encourage you to be more pessimistic in future, and to expect a life of tragedy, as a form of self-protection. I am a strong believer that this helps no one, and just means you are then faced with a life of less hope, of less peace and of less joy. I think it is a lot better to hold onto hope with both hands. To celebrate every ounce of happiness that lands in your lap, and to remain as positive as possible about the future. If you sadly need to face loss again, you deal with it then, but at least you have had seasons of glorious joy.

TASK FOR THE DAY

Have you become pessimistic about life? Write down two areas where your thoughts have focused on the negative, and then write down how you feel you could overcome that thinking.

1 _____

☞ I can overcome this thinking by

```

```

2 _____

☞ I can overcome this thinking by

```

```

✄ ✄

It shocks me how everyone assumes they know how
another should grieve. 'They should do it this way.'
'They are doing it wrong!' 'Why are they still weeping?'
So many questions, expectations and conflicting
opinions. There is only one truth, and that is this:

They are grieving their way and that is the
'only' right way.

✄ ✄ ✄ ✄ ✄ ✄ ✄ ✄ ✄ ✄ ZOË CLARK-COATES ✄ ✄ ✄ ✄ ✄ ✄ ✄ ✄ ✄ ✄

DAY 21

People used to tell me I was brave not to give up, but do you want to know the truth? I did; a hundred times a day, thousands of times a week, I gave up. I screamed, I yelled and sobbed, saying, 'That's it, I am done.' The pain overwhelmed me and I was fed up with being broken, down on my knees. So, if you are kicking yourself for giving up, please know this: *everyone* gives up. When the pain is all-consuming and life has lost its meaning, we all scream at the sky and shout, 'I can't take any more!' In that moment, we discover that life carries on regardless of whether we have the strength to continue or not, and all we need to do is sit for a while and wait for a fresh wave of courage to be bestowed upon us to refuel us for the next part of the journey.

TASK FOR THE DAY

There is something extremely cathartic in screaming at the sky, in shouting and releasing that internal pain. If you can find a place where you can go to scream, holler, wail and release some of the pain, do it today. You may also want to go to the gym and put on a pair of boxing gloves and hit a punch bag. Physical acts can truly help emotional pain.

When you have run out of tears and you are just left feeling empty and broken, this is when you need to search for the light. Even a fragment of sunshine will enable you to find those pieces of your broken heart lying on the floor. Slowly gather them, and your journey of healing will have begun.

ZOË CLARK-COATES

DAY 22

People often say, 'You will conquer this grief', as if it's an obstacle course you have to pole-vault over. But no one conquers grief, it is something you have to face, not fight; it can't be skipped over and it can't be defeated. You have to allow it to surround you like fog on a mountain top, and only when the fog rises can you see the path in front of you. It is not the enemy, even though it often feels like it. It is most certainly a giant – but it's a giant made out of love, pain, lessons, gentleness and a million other emotions. If we welcome the giant around the table, and don't try to make it stay on the other side of the door, it can teach us so much about ourselves and the world.

TASK FOR THE DAY

How would you describe grief? What does this giant look like in your life?

I expected to miss you in those silent solitary moments and I knew it would haunt me through the dark hours of the night. What I didn't expect was that the pain would have the ability to knock me off my feet while I was at a party, when I was laughing with friends, when I was enjoying a meal with family. Nothing prepares you for the power of grief.

ZOË CLARK-COATES

DAY 23

Who looked into your eyes and whispered in your ear that you are not enough? Who told you that you were responsible for this pain? Was it a family member? Was it a friend? Was it society? Or perhaps it was yourself? Whoever it was, they were not telling you the truth.

- You are enough.
- You are not responsible for this pain.
- You are worthy of love.
- You deserve to be praised and cared for.
- You do not need to keep your wounds hidden any longer, my friend.

Bravely show them to the world and let them heal.

TASK FOR THE DAY

Write a letter to yourself, telling yourself why you are strong, and why you are proud of yourself. You can empower yourself to move forwards. Be your own cheerleader.

Dear me,

There are a million things I want
to tell you, but the most important of all is:
'I will always love you.'

ZOË CLARK-COATES

DAY 24

Society often tells us that if something is common, we should accept it and not be overly bothered by it. People often used to remind me how common loss is, as if that would make me feel better. While it was nice to know I wasn't the only person in the world going through the agony of loss, knowing others were battling grief didn't make my pain any less; it just made me acutely aware of how many broken-hearted people were walking on this planet.

It is strange how people like to minimise pain, but I want to assure you that even if those around you don't acknowledge the gravity of your loss, I do. I know you are broken right now. I know no words I can offer will take that pain away from you. But sometimes it is enough to know our pain has been seen, and our loss has been recognised.

TASK FOR THE DAY

I want you to fill this box with all the words you feel right now. Write them simply, or write them in different sizes and different colours.

I had seen others journey through loss, I had read the books, I thought I understood it. But all the knowledge in the world, and all the preparation you can ever do, won't ever prepare you for how losing a loved one feels. I had heard the word 'broken' used, and I couldn't quite understand what that meant . . . until I broke. It is when the world seems black, devoid of hope, and you pray it stops spinning so you can get off. All-consuming pain with no respite. That is what it means to be broken.

ZOË CLARK-COATES

DAY 25

'What do you need?' I was asked this so many times when walking through grief. I often had no clue what I needed; my mind was overwhelmed and flooded with emotion. Sometimes I felt utterly numb, at other times a million different emotions consumed me. There were many occasions when I couldn't have conducted a conversation, but I still wanted to be with people, as I felt so lost and scared by the feelings I was trying to process. At those times I was only capable of sitting and staring at the wall, and I just needed someone to sit and stare at the wall with me. I wish I had been able to tell people that.

TASK FOR THE DAY

Think about what you need. If you can't find the words in the moment, perhaps take some time to write it down, and then give it to your friends and family to read. It can be incredibly hard to support someone through grief, and just giving people some pointers can be a huge help to them, but also to yourself down the line.

People often think those who have been through trauma and loss are more vulnerable, but they couldn't be more wrong. Those who have walked through the fire come out as warriors and are the best equipped to throw water on the flames surrounding others.

ZOË CLARK-COATES

DAY 26

What is your most difficult time each day? Mine was definitely the silent hours between 1am and 6am. These were the hours when grief consumed me and drained the room of all oxygen. When it became hard to breathe and surviving the loss seemed incomprehensible. Daylight seemed elusive and the birds were not even tempted to sing. I would often doubt that I could survive those nights, but I did, and you too will survive your haunting hours. Hold on, my friend. The sun will rise and hope will return.

TASK FOR THE DAY

Take 15 minutes to do something just for you. Whether it be reading a book, soaking in the bath, enjoying a coffee while looking at your garden – whatever you choose to do today, these minutes are your minutes and I hope they bring a smile to your face.

✎ ✎

To be told they had died was incomprehensible.
To continue living when my world was lying shattered at my feet was unthinkable. But I survived it and I promise you, my friend, you will survive it too.

✎ ✎ ✎ ✎ ✎ ✎ ✎ ✎ ✎ ZOË CLARK-COATES ✎ ✎ ✎ ✎ ✎ ✎ ✎ ✎ ✎ ✎

DAY 27

Where is your comfort zone? Perhaps you don't have one at all, or maybe you have two or three. My safe places were my bedroom, and especially my bathroom. As soon as I went into my bathroom and locked the door, I felt I could be totally real about the pain I was experiencing. I would kneel in my shower sobbing, but it felt so healing to just be free to be me. For some their safe place is sitting on a particular bench looking out to sea, for others it's in their car. So how long should someone reside in their comfort zone? Is it okay for people to sit in their safe place for months on end with little interaction with the outside world? Of course it's okay; whatever they need to do to survive is 100 per cent fine. I find that if people are comfortable publicly showing their pain and tears, they often retreat for shorter periods of time than those who struggle with showing their pain to the world, but there is no right and no wrong here. For those who are supporting the bereaved my best advice is this: Try to make all places safe places and all environments comfortable for the bereaved, by creating a culture of acceptance, love and vulnerability.

TASK FOR THE DAY

What are the thoughts that haunt you? Write them down. Once these emotions are expressed or verbalised, they can at times dissipate, as they are just seeking to be heard.

I think it is easy to fall into the mind-set that life is always trying to teach us something. I know when I was encountering deep loss I would scream to the heavens and say, 'Haven't I learnt the lesson yet? Do I really need to encounter more pain?' This is when I discovered loss isn't sent to punish us, to teach us, to transform us. It is just part of life, we have to experience it all, see it all – and to feel all the joy, we need to also feel all the pain.

ZOË CLARK-COATES

DAY 28

Grief has so many layers. After losing a loved one, it is obvious that a person will be grieving for the person they have lost, but it may surprise you that they will also be grieving over many other things simultaneously. One of the big things I grieved over was losing my joy. One day I was beyond happy, the next day I was beyond crushed, and I couldn't even imagine a time when I would smile again. I grieved for the fact I no longer cared about normal everyday things. Loss made these simple things feel irrelevant, even though they had previously brought me such joy. These are just a few of the things I mourned.

TASK FOR THE DAY

What are you grieving for besides the loss of your loved one?

1 _____

2 _____

3 _____

4 _____

Be patient.

Give yourself time to heal.

Rebuilding yourself following heartbreak is a slow process and it is something that can't be rushed.

So stop. Breathe. Wait.

ZOË CLARK-COATES

DAY 29

The silent scream. Only those who have ever produced this soul-churning scream will know what it is. When you fall to your knees and a silent scream leaves your lips, but there is no sound at all to be heard in this earthly realm. (I do wonder if it can perhaps be heard in another place? Perhaps heaven?) For me, the scream stopped once the shock passed; for others, I know the silent scream is ongoing and they believe it will never stop. One thing I can promise you is this: if your scream remains, you will learn to navigate around it, and in time you will get used to that holler humming in the background.

TASK FOR THE DAY

What would you tell someone who has just lost a loved one? What advice would you give them?

I didn't think I could survive pain like that. Before experiencing the heartache, I presumed I would crumble. While journeying it, I thought I might die from grief. In the weeks that followed, I assumed I would be broken forever. So I learnt a valuable lesson – I can and did survive the unimaginable and you will too.

ZOË CLARK-COATES

DAY 30

People kept asking me if I was ready. Ready to move forwards. How do you ever feel ready? What does feeling ready even mean? Does it mean we feel brave? Does it mean we feel sure and confident? If that is the case, I rarely feel ready for anything. What I have learnt on my journey is this: waiting to feel ready stops people from achieving their life goals. We just have to step forwards terrified. Heart racing. Hands shaking. Lip quivering. Stomach churning. And once we reach our end goal we can finally see – feeling ready is simply a myth.

TASK FOR THE DAY

What have you been postponing until you feel ready? Do you think you could take a chance and just move forwards? Now may not be the right time, of course, but perhaps it is? Maybe you just need to bravely step out of your comfort zone.

I used to grieve for the old me . . . the naive, innocent-to-loss me. The me that presumed a story would always end well. But then the light went on, the revelation took place – I liked this new me more.

The pain I had walked through made me kinder, deeper, truer and more empathetic. This was an enormous lesson to me; it showed me that good things can still grow in the darkest of places.

ZOË CLARK-COATES

DAY 31

I was so blessed to have my soulmate Andy by my side through loss, but so many people have to grieve with little or no support. If you can't share the pain and emotions you are experiencing with someone who empathises, you can quickly feel lost and isolated. I wanted everyone around me to comprehend that my world had stopped spinning. This is how I felt:

You died but still . . . the dawn breaks. The seas roar. The birds soar. The butterflies dance. The lightning strikes. The stars shine. The seasons fade. The earth spins. The icecaps thaw. The sun sets. But . . . my heart breaks. My soul cries. My eyes weep. My arms ache. My joy sleeps.

But how does anyone communicate this? And perhaps more importantly, how can we ensure those around us understand this? One way is by writing down how we feel, perhaps in letter form so we can carefully articulate the journey of loss.

TASK FOR THE DAY

Write your own letter to a loved one or a friend. Think of the things you want to say, that you may never have thought to express.

※ ※

I want to tell every person in the whole world
about you. I want the moon to know how I love you.
The stars to know how I adore you. The sun to
know how I will always miss you.

※ ※ ※ ※ ※ ※ ※ ※ ※ ※ ZOË CLARK-COATES ※ ※ ※ ※ ※ ※ ※ ※ ※ ※

DAY 32

It is common to fear being defined by the circumstances you have lived through, and if this becomes an over-whelming worry it is easy to change the dialogue used. I want to encourage you to stick with the fearless truth of your story, and not to worry about how society may see you. Don't get me wrong – I was concerned about this too, but along the way I learnt that most people don't look at those who talk of their pain and vulnerabilities through pity spectacles; they look at people with respect. When we open up our hearts and souls to the world, people want to come closer, they don't run in the opposite direction (well, authentic folk don't). People crave honesty, they long to see individuals displaying true sincerity, so please don't let fear rob you of speaking your authentic truth.

TASK FOR THE DAY

Write down exactly how you feel today, then pluck up the courage to tell someone what you have written.

When . . .

When . . . you find it hard to remember
the last time you looked forward to something.

When . . . you don't remember a time when you
weren't consumed with pain.

This is the time 'when' you need to hold on.

When . . . you need to trust life will get easier.

When . . . you need to believe broken hearts can heal.

When . . . you need to trust that tomorrow
could possibly be 'when'.

ZOË CLARK-COATES

DAY 33

I think most people who go through loss will tell you that when people around you are complaining about their partner coming in late, or moaning about something you would now give anything to have, it kind of grates. The temptation when you hear someone saying, 'Wow, I had a tough night with my partner snoring' is to yell, 'Do you know what I would give to be kept up all night by my partner?!' Of course, I wouldn't encourage you to say this to anyone, but I wanted to include it here to show you that you aren't alone if you are feeling this right now. While we often need to hold our tongues in these moments, resentment/irritation can sneakily creep up on us. The best way to process these feelings is to talk about them with a safe person (i.e. someone who would not report it back to the person saying it), as just by verbalising the frustration it can help diminish or eliminate the feelings you are experiencing.

TASK FOR THE DAY

Write a list of the things you are struggling to hear and deal with. Once you have written the list, consider how you could respond in a kind way, to change the future dialogue.

I can always recognise those who have been broken.
For they now carry a light – a light that can only be
bestowed on those who have been shattered
by heartbreak.

They are filled with greater levels of compassion,
of empathy and of kindness, for they know first-hand
what true pain feels like.

ZOË CLARK-COATES

DAY 34

Anniversaries and occasions.

For some, these are dates to look forward to, as those around them join them in talking about the one they have lost; for others, the days bring a fresh wave of grief and can make the feelings of isolation seem suffocating. Others don't mark any dates in the diary and the days pass without notice. I fall into this last category: I chose not to carve out any dates in my calendar; perhaps that's because I have had repeated loss, and there would be too many dates to circle, but it could also be because I made a conscious choice to celebrate and talk about the ones I have lost 365 days a year, and that meant I didn't feel a need to have set days each year to process pain or celebrate them. However, for some these dates will forever be ingrained and they have no choice but to acknowledge them in their lives. So, what do I suggest to people to help them get through birth or death anniversaries, Mother's and Father's Day, wedding anniversaries etc.? I always recommend they find something they love to do to mark these dates. Perhaps that's a walk in the park, maybe it's planting a new plant or tree, maybe it's going to a lovely café and having a slice of their favourite cake – but do something that makes you smile, as that means you can remember your loved one with a smile. Don't get me wrong – you may need to weep a river on those days and that's okay; it's a grief layer being processed. But if you can also do something you enjoy, it can help with the agony of the day.

TASK FOR THE DAY

What do you love to do? Can you think of something you could do yearly to celebrate the person you have lost if you do want to mark the dates on your calendar?

Write your ideas here:

Talk about it. Then talk some more. Then a little more.

The story you hold deep in your heart wants
to be told – needs to be told.

It is in the telling. It is in the sharing.

It is in the revealing of your soul that the healing begins.

ZOË CLARK-COATES

DAY 35

It is very common post-loss to feel you are spending your life apologising for things that just flew out of your mouth. Grief seems to remove a filter, and without even meaning to be rude you may have found yourself saying the most awful things to the people around you. People often say to me, 'Maybe it would be easier if I walked around with a sign saying "I'm sorry", as I seem to offend people without even trying.' So if you feel this, know you are not alone. When you are trying to process pain and deal with profound loss, it is very difficult to control your emotions and your tongue, and one of the horrible side effects of this is sadly putting your foot in it on a regular basis. So just be honest, be willing to apologise, and ask for grace from the people who love you.

TASK FOR THE DAY

Tell your story here (if you need more space, write your story elsewhere and use this space for thoughts):

If today you are hurting. If tomorrow you are weeping.
That is okay. My friend, your heart is just healing.

ZOË CLARK-COATES

DAY 36

Loss divides your life into before and after.

Nothing looks or feels the same post-loss. Why is this? I believe it is because you change as a person so radically once you have walked through profound grief that the world seems very different. It's like you have stepped through a door you never knew was there, and that door was firmly locked behind you as you went through it. There is no return to the old you, or that past world, and this is why life divides into before and after. While this can be traumatising and something in itself to grieve for, it can also be liberating. You now have the chance to recreate how you want the world to look. It's a blank piece of paper. Yes, it may be soggy with tears for some time, but it's still blank. Maybe it's time to make new friends? Maybe it's time to consider a change of direction with your career? Perhaps it's time to start a new hobby? When I made these changes in my life, they felt like gifts from my children, like they were gifting me additional levels of happiness. Loss doesn't need only to bring heartbreak; your loved one can also bring you beautiful, life-changing gifts.

TASK FOR THE DAY

Consider what gifts your loved one has brought or could still bring you to make your life better:

1 _____

2 _____

3 _____

4 _____

5 _____

Where does hope rest? I guess it's different in every person, but everyone can find their source. Search for that place in your soul where happiness once sat comfortably next to peace. Where your sense of purpose drove you forwards, and fear couldn't even stop you facing giants. In that secret place is your reserve of hope, and once it's rediscovered a journey can begin.

ZOË CLARK-COATES

DAY 37

There is no hierarchy in grief.

The world often tells us that loss past x point is worse than at y point. Or a child you lose at x age is worse than losing a child aged y. I find this extraordinarily hard to understand and refuse to accept it, and will spend my life fighting this utterly wrong belief. Loss is loss. Grief is grief. Someone's age doesn't denote their worth, their place in this world or the significance of them as a person. Likewise, the time you have spent with a person doesn't dictate the length of the grieving process you are allowed to have after their passing.

No one has the right to diminish your grief or your pain, or tell you how your loss was less important or notable than another's. There is simply no hierarchy in grief and, if we can collectively use our voices to say this, I think we will become a better, more compassionate society, one that supports without prejudice anyone who is hurting.

TASK FOR THE DAY

Use this space to write down the misconceptions you feel surround your loss.

Your time on earth was not as long as I would have
hoped. But you were the plot changer. The colour giver.
The character builder. The joy bringer. Once you entered
my life, no page was ever the same again

ZOË CLARK-COATES

DAY 38

Good and bad care post-loss.

How you are treated when you are going through loss makes the world of difference in how you process the pain and trauma attached to loss. If you or your loved one received poor care, I can only say how sorry I am, as everyone should be treated with true compassion when journeying through one of the most traumatic life events. If you received excellent care, I am so pleased, and I know you will be able to speak of how empathy and kindness made your experience so much easier.

So, what do we do if we didn't witness or experience good care? We speak about it. We write to the GP, hospital, or to whoever fell below our expected standard. Now, I know this is easy to say and hard to do, but it's only when we speak out and hold people to account that things change. And, yes, I know it won't bring your loved one back, and it may feel pointless in the scheme of things; but it isn't pointless, it will make a difference, so please take 20 minutes to write about your experience.

What do you do if there was great care? Speak about it and also write to the people who provided that care. When we take the time to offer praise and gratitude to caregivers, it makes them feel appreciated, but just as importantly it encourages good practice. So please thank and praise all who excelled in their care and compassion.

TASK FOR THE DAY

Write to the care-givers and tell them about the great, or poor, care.

~~~~~~

Sometimes people just need time.

Time to sit.

Time to just 'be' with the pain.

Time to let the tears pool.

Time to let the heart mend.

Time to accept life will never be the same again.

The issue for many?

They are rarely given 'time'.

~~~~~~~~~ ZOË CLARK-COATES ~~~~~~~~~

DAY 39

What do you do when you can't face another day, when the pain is too overwhelming? You have two choices: you can either try to run from it, which I can tell you now is pretty hard to do, and nine times out of ten it will chase after you and will eventually catch you when you least expect it; or you yield to the pain. You dive in; you lie on the floor and let the pain surround you. You don't fight the tears, you let those body-shaking sobs consume your soul. You throw down your armour and say, 'I will no longer battle with these emotions, I surrender.'

When we surrender, we let grief take us to the next level. The tears transport us to somewhere new. It takes real courage to face pain like this head-on, so believe me when I say I am not trying to make this sound simple and easy. It's heartbreaking and possibly one of the toughest things one can do in this life – but by doing it you will be helping yourself in the long term.

TASK FOR THE DAY

Are you ready to take off your armour and lay down your sword? Will you just look pain in the eye and say, 'I will not run from you. I will simply let it flow through me and transform me as it runs through my veins.' If you are ready to do this, try this exercise:

Lie on the floor and clench every muscle in your body.

Screw up your face into a grimace and squeeze your hands into tight fists. Think of the emotional pain you are carrying. Hold for five seconds and then release fully. As you release, imagine yourself removing the armour you have been wearing and let the tears flow.

I find it helps to play music loudly when doing this. My song of choice is 'Hallelujah' by Jeff Buckley.

Please know that this exercise can be exhausting emotionally, so don't do it just before leaving for work or an event. Take a few hours afterwards to regroup and to relax.

We are less without you as part of us is missing.
Yet we are more ourselves than ever before,
as your existence made us explore our souls.

This is the dichotomy of loss.

ZOË CLARK-COATES

DAY 40

How often have we been told not to cry, or perhaps how many times have we told others not to cry? Society doesn't allow much space for weeping; we have been taught wrongly that to be strong means showing no or very little emotion. Yes, of course we can accept the odd pretty tear falling down a person's cheek, and may even be touched at seeing it before us, but it's different if someone is sobbing hysterically at our feet. If we are the one weeping, it feels messy, ugly and out of control. If we are the ones witnessing it, it can make us feel helpless and inept at dealing with such visible distress. But this is where we have gone wrong as humans. Emotion, *all* emotion is what makes us human; we should welcome the heart-wrenching sobs as much as we welcome the belly-doubling hysterical laughs. Life is amazing, but it can also be utterly crap. It can be beautiful and so very ugly. It can bring unending joy and endless pain. But we survive it by embracing every moment, by allowing ourselves and others to express it all – whether that be by weeping an ocean of tears, or by laughing till tears of joy roll down our cheeks.

TASK FOR THE DAY

Let the tears roll. Tears of grief and sadness are made of a different substance from tears of joy – how amazing is that? They contain hormones and chemicals, and it is essential we let them out so they can't cause damage to us emotionally and/or physically. So be kind to yourself and let them flow today. It may help to put on a piece of music, or go into the shower . . .

You have so much more life to experience.

More love. More pain. More joy. More suffering.

Grasp everything with two hands.

Feel it all.

It is only when we embrace both the dark
and the light that we can live an extraordinary life.

ZOË CLARK-COATES

DAY 41

How can you let go of someone or something you have wanted so much? I wish there was a skill to make this easier, but sadly there isn't. It will never be easy letting go of a person you have loved dearly, but equally I don't think it should be easy. It should be gut-wrenching, it should be a battle, it should tear our hearts apart. Loss should be incomprehensible and bring us to our knees. The pain reveals the love. And while we have to let go physically of the person, they will never leave our hearts, our minds, our lives. All those we have loved and lost remain on the pages of our books forever.

TASK FOR THE DAY

Saying goodbye to a person's physical body is so incredibly hard. Maybe for you that will take place at a funeral; perhaps it is on a hillside as you scatter the ashes of the one you adore. Wherever and whenever it is, it will be a moment that lives with you forever. To come to terms with that process, I want to encourage you to talk about the event. By talking about it, you allow your brain to accept what has happened and eventually, over time, you may gain a deeper level of peace.

As I resurfaced from the blackest part of grief,
I quickly learnt I should stop seeking the big moments.
You know, those moments you crave with the same
desperation as a person crawling in the desert
seeking water. Moments that feel so elusive
and unreachable, like . . .

Feeling total peace in your soul.
Feeling excited about the year ahead.
Not being consumed with pain.
Not fearing tears could spontaneously
spring from your eyes.

Instead, I needed to look towards the little moments . . .

The smile that broke forth without
any warning when something amused me.
The kindness of a stranger who asked me how I was.
The taste of that sweet peach that was nurtured
and grown for me to enjoy.
The joy I felt seeing my friend get their wish granted.

And this is how my journey changed.
I learnt that life could be all kinds of wonderful
just by appreciating the little moments.

ZOË CLARK-COATES

DAY 42

Feeling guilt over grieving is super-common. It is hard to carry grief when we feel guilt for bringing sadness to the table. If all those present want to just be happy and look at the brighter side of life, and then you come along with swollen eyes and tear-soaked tissues, whatever is or isn't said, you can quickly feel awful for changing the tone of the conversation or for lowering the positive energy. Over time this guilt can build and most bereaved people will withdraw themselves from the table, or even the house, because the weight of the guilt on top of the grief is just too much. If you are the bereaved person, I want to encourage you to fight this guilt and show up anyway. This urge to protect others can at times magnify your pain, and however much we want to conceal sadness from our loved ones, we are robbing them from seeing the full expanse of life, which is essential to authentic living. For those who are supporting the heartbroken and are sitting around that table, I urge you to constantly reassure the bereaved that it's okay to bring their tears and pain to every meal, make them know it's a safe place, and no guilt is needed, as this will help them on their walk to healing.

TASK FOR THE DAY

Are you carrying guilt? List the things you feel guilty about, and then decide how you can lay down that guilt and walk into freedom.

1 _____

2 _____

3 _____

4 _____

5 _____

There will be days where you are hit by a fresh wave of grief and you will doubt how far you have swum in the ocean of mourning. Let me reassure you that these waves are part of the journey, they won't put you back. In fact, they do the exact opposite; they carry you forwards if you don't fight them – just hold onto your life ring and let the current carry you on. You won't drown, but you may need to tell yourself this a hundred times a day. Let it become your mantra: 'I won't drown; I am just learning to swim.'

ZOË CLARK-COATES

DAY 43

Wanting to protect others.

It is so normal to want to protect those around us from the pain we ourselves are walking, so if you are feeling this, please know you are not alone. I often used to say I was fine to family members as I couldn't cope with them crying, and that was for two reasons. Firstly, I didn't want them to be in pain; but secondly, I felt so broken myself that having then to try to pick someone else up off the floor was something I simply couldn't handle, physically or mentally. The issue with all of the above is that it stops you being real about what you are going through. At some point, you have to draw a line and say, firstly, 'I can't protect others from the pain of loss, and, if I try to, I am actually robbing them of the chance to process their grief.' Secondly, people don't expect the grieving person to help them, so it is okay to stand back and say, 'It hurts, doesn't it?' This is then a time for you all to cry together, and not a time for you to become the superhero and save them from the grief.

TASK FOR THE DAY

Consider whether you are trying to rescue people from grief. Just as they can't save you from this pain, you can't rescue them either. Choose to be real in all circumstances, even if that means a friend or family member regularly sharing tears with you. Those who grieve together heal together.

*　*

And then, one cloudy afternoon, I decided it was time. It was time to lay down my sword. To stop fighting the pain. To give up the relentless battle not to cry. I fully submitted. I looked into the eyes of suffering and declared, 'I can do this. I will not run from you, grief. I will give you the space you deserve.'

And that, my friend, is when my healing began.

*　*　*　*　*　*　*　* ZOË CLARK-COATES *　*　*　*　*　*　*　*

DAY 44

Tears have a voice. Pain has a voice. How often do we refuse to let that voice be heard, though? We just silence it and refuse to give it a time to talk. We learn so much about ourselves and the experience we have walked through if we do give tears and pain space to communicate.

At times my tears screamed of physical agony; at other times they spoke of desperation, of heartbreak, of fear and of dread. Grief and loss are so utterly confusing. A million emotions and a trillion feelings, and all of them are connected to this tiny, five-letter word called grief.

TASK FOR THE DAY

Write in the tear shapes below some of the key things your tears are trying to communicate.

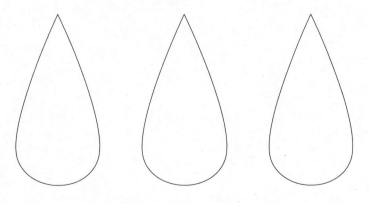

The world tells us it is good to be strong, it is great to be fearless. It feeds us messages that being broken is weakness and tears are self-indulgent. We are patted on the back if 'we held it together', and are awarded a badge of bravery if we manage to fake a smile through the pain. I long for the day when as a community we say enough. When we stand as one and say expressing human emotion is what makes us human. To show one's scars and to reveal hidden pain is heroic.

Vulnerability is beautiful and, once society embraces this, we will give all people permission to be real . . . to be them.

ZOË CLARK-COATES

DAY 45

Impending loss.

One of the hardest things for me to live through was impending loss. Time went so slowly; every day felt like a year and emotionally I was on a terrifying rollercoaster. One moment I was trying to believe everything would be okay, and the next second I was trying to prepare myself for the loss. I felt guilty for even considering they might not make it, and I felt ridiculous for daring to hope they might be okay. During this time, emotions adjust to being on high alert and adrenaline pumps through your veins 24/7. Post-loss, this doesn't simply cease, as your body has grown accustomed to living in what has felt like dangerous terrain, so as well as processing the grief, you also need to reprogramme your mind and let it learn to rest again, and allow for this fight-or-flight response to settle.

TASK FOR THE DAY

How do we reprogramme our mind and give it time to adjust if it has been in a state of high alert for some time?

Firstly, talk, and keep talking so the brain can get to grips with the emotional turmoil you have had to process. Secondly, you need to find something to help you relax. This may be exercise, it may be relaxation therapy, it may be reading, but it needs to be something that lets your mind be calm and ideally gives you time off from thinking. We live in a world where stillness is hard to find; now is a time you need to seek it out and learn to stand still, breathe deeply and slow your heart rate. Try to do this today and every day going forwards.

Some days it hurts from nowhere.

One moment the sun is shining through the window, which is making you smile, the next moment the grief consumes you like a tornado. It lifts you up and throws you into a heap of tears on the floor.

Grief is the ultimate force. A presence that needs no invite, it just enters the room whenever it pleases. This is why we need to respect it and to honour it.

It will journey with you now for life, and only you can choose whether it is the enemy or a reluctant companion.

ZOË CLARK-COATES

DAY 46

My loved one was robbed of all their tomorrows, but because of them I embrace all of my todays – and you can too. This isn't me saying look on the bright side; it's me purely saying that in all of this pain, in all of this broken-ness, the people who have gone before us can offer us beautiful gifts. And one of these gifts is an appreciation of life and a tangible sense of the fragility of life, which can make you seize every joy-filled moment with two hands. For a long time, I couldn't feel anything but pain, but, as time went on, I became aware of these beautiful gifts.

TASK FOR THE DAY

Do you feel in a place where you can see the gifts your loved one brought you? If you do, list them below. If you can't see them as yet, list below the gifts you hope they will bring.

1 _____

2 _____

3 _____

4 _____

5 _____

6 _____

7 _____

As humans we crave connection.
We plead for compassion, and the most profound
gift we can ever receive is to be understood . . .
And there is no greater time to be handed that
gift than when one is grieving.

ZOË CLARK-COATES

DAY 47

If yesterday you ran from the pain . . . but today you sit with the pain . . . and tomorrow you face the pain . . . that, my friend, is the journey to healing a broken heart.

So please don't panic. Please don't feel you should be further along the path than you currently are.

You are doing fine. You don't need to walk at someone else's speed. You don't need to fret if people make you feel you are healing too slowly; that is their issue, not yours.

Your loss.

Your pain.

Your walk.

TASK FOR THE DAY

Write a letter to yourself pre-loss, giving yourself your best tips for how to navigate loss. Then look at that letter – are you now following your own advice?

> *Dear me,*

When you are bereft and you find someone who speaks the language of grief, it feels like 'home'.

ZOË CLARK-COATES

DAY 48

Have you ever cried for so long you are scared? Scared you will never stop weeping? Scared that this is how life will look forever? Scared that you will never smile again?

This fear is so normal and it is okay to acknowledge it, and it helps to discuss it.

When grief grips your soul, it feels bleak and desolate, and this lack of hope for a brighter tomorrow is part of the grieving process.

I promise you the sun will rise and this scary, black grief will lessen.

Try not to even consider what tomorrow has in store when you feel the terror take hold; just focus on today. If today seems too much to handle, just get through the next hour. Whether you take massive steps forwards, or the tiniest micro steps, it doesn't matter; progress is being made – and you, my friend, are going to make it through.

TASK FOR THE DAY

Write down in these steps the six things you can do to help you get through today.

Some of you spent last night searching for fragments of your broken heart. Others sat in shock as their heart felt like it had imploded. Each day now feels like a year; and when you are told to just survive the next hour, you want to scream, as 60 more minutes of this pain feels like torture. So, let me tell you this: it's okay to stop surviving, it's okay to just stay on the floor. It's okay to say, 'This hurts', it's okay not to know how you will live beyond this day. This is black grief, this is surreal grief, and I promise you it will lift. Perhaps it won't lift today, and maybe not tomorrow, but one day the black grief will turn to grey, and you will survive.

ZOË CLARK-COATES

DAY 49

Broken hearts continue to beat.

Now I see this as a good thing, but when I was broken it was the last thing I wanted to hear. I didn't want my heart to carry on beating, I wanted to be saved from the pain. So if that's how you feel today, I want you to know that I get it, I hear your pain.

There is a phrase commonly bandied about that I used to hate with a passion, and that is: 'time heals all wounds'. Is it correct? No, time doesn't automatically heal all wounds, but it is possible for the wounds to no longer bleed. And, yes, that does happen over time and can't be fast-forwarded. So, while I wish I could point you in the direction of a secret trap door that fast-forwards time for you, I sadly can't, and I just hope you can believe me when I say this . . .

It will get easier.

You are going to make it through this black tunnel.

Just hold on.

TASK FOR THE DAY

Find something to distract you for 15 minutes today. It could be listening to a piece of music you adore that has lots of happy memories attached to it, or losing yourself in a good movie. You can think of anything but loss and pain – this is your 15 minutes to escape.

Not everyone stays forever.
Some people arrive, change us and then leave.
How we continue on once they have departed is
what shows the world they were ever
here at all.

ZOË CLARK-COATES

DAY 50

Oh, how I wish the world would recognise and acknowledge that one person can never replace another. Also, grieving in no way shows a lack of gratitude for another living soul. Pain and joy, tears and smiles, even regret and thankfulness can easily sit alongside one another, so don't let anyone tell you any different, my friend.

You can feel it all . . . In the same hour you can scream and laugh. You can feel helpless and hopeful. You can want to die and want to live.

This is what grieving looks like: a consortium of opposing feelings in one mind, in one body. You are normal to feel it all.

TASK FOR THE DAY

How would you describe your grief today?

If you start questioning, 'Why me?',
you can end up feeling like a victim. Flipping that
question on its head and saying, 'Why not me?'
can help you rise to the battle at hand.

ZOË CLARK-COATES

DAY 51

Loss is made up of 'if onlys'. If only I held you longer. If only I called you more often. If only I had spent more quality time with you.

I used to constantly ask myself how I could console myself, knowing that the millions of questions or regrets I have will never be answered or rectified? I thought I was destined to live in turmoil and internal conflict, but I was wrong. I found peace with not knowing and peace with knowing I can't change the past. That doesn't mean I still wouldn't love to know all the answers; it just means I learnt to accept that I can't know.

There wasn't a magical moment when this peace arrived, and it wasn't something I did that made it happen. Over time I just gradually became accustomed to living with the unknowns and accepting the past can't be altered, and that brought with it a feeling of being okay to live with a million question marks and an acceptance that I did the best I could with the time I was given.

I hope if you wrestle with questions and internal conflict that one day you too will find peace.

TASK FOR THE DAY

In what areas of your life would you like to feel more peace?

Is there anything you can do to get that peace? If there is, consider doing it . . .

Your story. Your pain. Your loss.
All of it, every single part of it, deserves to be heard.
Deserves to be recognised.
Deserves to be given time to heal.

ZOË CLARK-COATES

DAY 52

When we are young, we are taught how to articulate joy and happiness but we are rarely taught the language of loss. How do you even begin to express earth-shattering pain? Loss flings you into a world of medical terminology, and while trying to translate that you are simultaneously expected to explain to those around you the depth of heartache you are experiencing. I just wanted people to understand that my world was unravelling in front of my eyes, and however much I begged for the pain to stop, it didn't. But I couldn't find the words in my fog of grief to tell them anything other than, 'I am hurting.'

TASK FOR THE DAY

What are you struggling to express to those around you?
Use this space to try to verbalise what you would want the
world to know.

Just because someone isn't publicly weeping,
doesn't mean their heart isn't privately breaking.

ZOË CLARK-COATES

DAY 53

My soul seemed to know what to do to survive . . . it wanted to talk, to explain, to express, to verbalise the agony my heart was trying to process. My mind, on the other hand, wanted me to be silent, to not risk more pain – to share means to be vulnerable, and when you reveal the heartache you have suffered, you in turn invite comments from those who hear your story. So, the mission is to be guided by your soul, while quietening your thoughts, so your heart can start to mend.

I looked for people who inspired me to step out. I needed to be encouraged to voice my story and I encourage you to do the same.

TASK FOR THE DAY

Who inspires you and why? Even by considering this question you are looking beyond the superficial and looking deep. The people we often admire and respect don't have it all together; they are the people who are real about life.

When you fear you can't handle another day on
this planet, just remind yourself you can and you will.
Your heart can't even comprehend the hidden
strength your mind holds.

ZOË CLARK-COATES

DAY 54

Every once in a while, we discover a person who changes our perspective on life. They fearlessly and perhaps even without knowing it guide us on our personal journey. They make us smile, but will just as happily sit with us as we shed a million tears. These people are sacred, and we won't meet many of them on our walk through life, so cherish them, hold them close and treat them with love, as they will be a lamp in the darkness.

TASK FOR THE DAY

Friends and family can transform our experience of loss, and take it from being one of isolation to one filled with love. Who are the friends who have helped you survive your journey of loss? Has any friend surprised you with their kindness?

Friends who have helped me

Oh, just to sit by you, one more time,
and to hold your hand, what a gift that would be.

ZOË CLARK-COATES

DAY 55

What makes people tired when they are grieving? Is it the lack of hope that makes them so weary? Is it the immense pain they are carrying in their heart that weighs them down? Is it the dread of a new day bringing another 24 hours for them to face? Is it that grief robs them of deep and restful sleep as they are haunted by nightmares of loss? Whatever it is, grief is utterly exhausting. If you feel spent, broken, tired and don't know how you can even face today, trust me when I say your energy will return. My advice is to be selective in terms of what you choose to do, and use the energy you do have for basic survival, until strength returns to you.

TASK FOR THE DAY

Rest. This is your task. True rest if that is possible. Take a long shower, or lie in the bath and relax. Thirty minutes of doing nothing.

What do you love to do, but never have time for? Think how you can make time in your life to do this more.

I was so tired.
My heart was tired.
My brain was tired.
My tears were tired.
I begged to feel numb, so numb I could
sleep without nightmares.
Just 24 hours without feeling crippling pain in my heart.
But grief doesn't give you time off.
Not a day, not an hour, not even a crummy minute.
Grief doesn't care if you are tired.
Grief just wants to be felt.
Grief just wants to be heard.
This is why grieving is exhausting,
as there is no respite.

ZOË CLARK-COATES

DAY 56

What do you wish you had known about grief before experiencing it?

There are so many things I wished I had known. Firstly, I wish I had been aware that grief consumes you, every part of you, and it makes you feel lost and alone, but this feeling does pass. I was so scared when this happened to me, and if I had known the feelings wouldn't last forever that would have really helped me.

I wish I had known that I am not responsible for others' grief. I felt so guilty that our losses brought so much pain to other people's lives, so I tried to rescue them from that. I now wish I had just let them process their pain and not used my small energy reserves to protect them.

I wish I had known it was okay to smile, and by me smiling I wasn't in any way saying my loved ones' lives didn't matter. The fear of this held me back from laughing for so long.

TASK FOR THE DAY

What do you wish you had known?

1 _____

2 _____

3 _____

4 _____

5 _____

~ ~

If only loving someone meant they were guaranteed
to stay, how much sweeter would life be.

~ ~ ~ ~ ~ ~ ~ ~ ~ ZOË CLARK-COATES *~ ~ ~ ~ ~ ~ ~ ~ ~*

DAY 57

We are taught that grief has neat steps – I can almost laugh at that now. Oh, how simple it would be if we could have a tick list of grief stepping stones, where we carefully leap from one step to the next.

Grief isn't like that. This is what grief looks like:

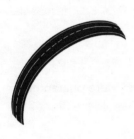

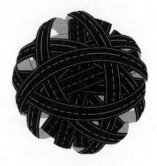

What people think the journey of grief looks like . . .

What it actually looks like

When we can accept that grief isn't linear, I think it truly helps our journey through loss, as most grieving people fear they have lost the plot. All their emotions have gone haywire and they have no clue what they will feel like minute by minute.

So, trust me when I say grief isn't neat; it's messy and it is hard and whether you are standing today, or lying on the floor weeping, you are doing fine.

TASK FOR THE DAY

Draw a picture of what your grief looks like:

People spend so much time trying to get back
to who they were pre-loss, and even if they got there
(which they can't) they would discover they no longer
belong in that world. The space they left is no
longer their shape. The only way to find the
new them is to move forwards.

ZOË CLARK-COATES

DAY 58

Surviving loss is like swimming in the ocean with no clue as to whether you can swim. You don't enter the water at the shore, you get dropped into the deepest part, and no land is even in sight. Waves often go over your head and you are convinced you will drown.

Then you see a lifebuoy and reach out to it, knowing it is your one chance of survival. You grab it with a very weak hand, and cling to it for dear life.

Only when strength has returned can you attempt to swim again. With fear and trepidation, you decide to attempt to reach dry land, and launch into the waves. As you discover you can in fact swim, you look to your left and then to your right, and that is when you see a host of other people swimming in the same direction.

You are not alone. Everyone has the same look of fear on their face, but together you are stronger. As one, you swim to land.

And that, my friend, is how you survive loss . . . Together. In unity. All terrified. All unsure about being able to swim. All afraid of the water.

But the strength of swimming in the same direction carries you through to land.

TASK FOR THE DAY

Find a piece of music that encourages you and makes you feel you do have the strength to make it to land.

One of my favourite songs which spurs me on is Whitney Houston's 'I Did Not Know My Own Strength'!

Oh, how I used to wish that I didn't feel
everything so intensely.

I longed to be a person who just experienced
things at a superficial level, where a simple sweep
of the hand would banish any hurt I felt.

But I wasn't that person. I felt it all. Deeply. Crushingly.
The pain was ceaseless. The grief was unyielding.

I had assumed that was my great weakness but
I couldn't have been more wrong, as this was actually
my superpower.

Because I felt it all, I had no choice but to embrace it,
to process it, and to allow it to change me.

Through the pain, I discovered who I was, and by
holding on to hope I found my purpose.

ZOË CLARK-COATES

DAY 59

Feeling lonely is horrific and most grief-stricken people will tell you that they feel desperately lonely. This happens for two reasons: firstly, because they have lost a person they love. Secondly, grieving is such a solitary experience and, when walking through grief, a person will often feel like they are the only person on the planet enduring the pain. I wish there was a magic cure – if there was, I would definitely hand it to you right now, as I would love to rescue everyone from feeling the pain of loneliness. There are a few tips I can offer, however. Firstly, if you are trying to get used to a silent house, consider how you can change this. For some people it helps to invite someone to live with them for a period of time; others find taking care of a pet brings an element of comfort. If neither of these things is possible, consider leaving music playing on the radio each day, just so you get to hear other voices. Call people daily on the phone so you have some personal interaction. Try to leave the house as often as possible – although it's agonising seeing that the planet has continued to turn while your world has imploded, it does make your integration into daily life easier in the long term.

TASK FOR THE DAY

What makes you feel lonely right now? Are there things that may help you deal with this?

While you remember them, they will live forever.

ZOË CLARK-COATES

DAY 60

I often wonder, when do friends become family? It is certainly not dictated by the length of the relationship, as some friends come into your life and within hours they are family. So what is it? Where, how and when does this magic happen? I believe it happens when your souls connect. Within minutes of the conversation starting, you can tell you are on the same wavelength. You feel instantly comfortable with sharing intimate truths and revealing hidden parts of your heart. You know they would be your 3am call should crisis strike, and your gut tells you that they would never ask, 'Why are you calling?'; they would just say, 'How can I help?' Forever friends . . . that is what they are called.

TASK FOR THE DAY

Who are your forever friends?

Are there others you feel you could become closer to? If yes, what could you do to make those relationships stronger?

Free yourself from wrong expectation.

There is no fixed time period in which the
darkest part of grief must pass.
There isn't a timeframe in which you must
smile or even function.
There is no worldly standard for what is 'normal'
when it comes to mourning a loved one.
This is a myth spun by those who don't know how
grief works – those lucky souls who have never been
on the receiving end of a life-changing loss.

So, however you feel today – that is normal.
However much you hurt – that is normal.
How much you cry – that is normal.
Your grief. Your loss. Your normal.

ZOË CLARK-COATES

Does that ache ever go, that deep longing
to be back with the one you have lost?

In my experience no,
it stays, it becomes part of your DNA.
You ache because you love them.
You miss them as they are irreplaceable.

But you learn to accept this new reality,
this new state of being, as the love you had and
will always have for them, is worth your
soul aching for eternity.

ZOË CLARK-COATES

Help and Resources

International support following baby loss

Advice, support, befriending, international remembrance services, counselling, support via social media and more.

The Mariposa Trust – Saying Goodbye is the primary division which offers support post-baby loss, but the charity has many other divisions too.

- mariposatrust.org
- sayinggoodbye.org

Marriage counselling and support

- relate.org.uk
- themarriagecourses.org/try/the-marriage-course/

Support for children who are grieving

- winstonswish.org
- youngminds.org.uk

Bereavement support and counselling

- mariposatrust.org
- soultears.org
- sayinggoodbye.org
- psychotherapy.org.uk/find-a-therapist/
- cruse.org.uk
- mind.org.uk
- nhs.uk/conditions/counselling/
- bacp.co.uk/search/Therapists
- acc-uk.org
- anxietyuk.org.uk
- counselling-directory.org.uk
- mindandsoulfoundation.org

Emotional support for people in distress

- Samaritans – samaritans.org
- SOBS – uksobs.org

Other useful contacts

- bereavementadvice.org
- nhs.uk
- mayoclinic.org

Thank You

Firstly thank you for reading this book, it takes huge trust and strength to read another's words when one is grieving, and I hope mine have brought you some comfort.

Thank you to all the individuals who contributed their stories to *Beyond Goodbye*. Thank you for trusting me with your words and allowing them to be included in this book, because of you people will feel less alone

Thanks to my agent Jane Graham-Maw, my publishers Orion Springs (especially Amanda Harris and Lucinda McNeile) and all those who left their fingerprints on this book, it is because of you *Beyond Goodbye* is now sitting on the shelves in the shops, rather than being just a file in my brain.

Thanks to my beautiful friend Ali Herbert for naming this book.

Thanks to all my family (especially my mum and dad, Sue and Richard Clark, and sister Hayley and brother-in-law Justin) and beautiful friends (you know who you are) who support and encourage me every step of the way, knowing you are in my corner makes all the difference and I love you dearly.

Thanks to my church leaders Tim and Rachel Hughes

and our whole church family, you championing us makes the world of difference. Making St Luke's, Gas Street our home church was one of the best life decisions we have made.

A special HUGE thank you to Andy, my husband, soul mate and biggest cheerleader – I only get to write as you create the time for me to do so, so thank you – You are my bestest friend, my heartbeat and I will love you forever.

To my two daughters Esme Emilia and Bronte Jemima, I promised you I would try to make a difference so you could reside in a more compassionate world, I hope I am doing you proud. You are world changers, light bringers, and are filled with endless joy. I pray that you will continue to dream big and will never forget you have the power in your hands to help those around you . . . I love you to the moon and back, thank you for being so utterly amazing.

To my five little ones who ran ahead – Cobi, Darcey, Bailey, Samuel and Isabella, enjoy playing on the streets of gold until Mama comes home to be with you.

My final words have to go to my grandfather, Raymond Samuel James McHale. You never got to hold this book in your hands, but my love for you is on every single page. Just a little of your story is shared here, and even a short interview I did with you . . . oh how I wish you could have contributed more and seen your words in print. I certainly never expected to be weeping tears of grief whilst completing it, I believed saying goodbye to you was another century away, and this is yet another reminder to me, to appreciate every moment one has with those we love.

Grandad, you always lent your copies of my books to everyone you knew, though this probably frustrated the book shops of Devon, due to the sales you lost them, I love how proud you were of my work and your heart to help others. I could say so much more, I feel the need to say so much more . . . but the bottom line comes down to this – I love you, I miss you and I so wish you were here – and this book is dedicated to you.

Legacy Scheme

If this book has helped you, would you consider purchasing copies to help others?

Maybe you would like to buy a couple of copies for friends or family who have lost, or perhaps you might like to purchase copies in bulk? Many people around the world have fundraised to enable them to buy hundreds of copies of my first book, *Saying Goodbye*, and second book *The Baby Loss Guide* in honour of the child they have lost. They then donate these books to hospitals, hospices, clinics, GP practices, churches or support groups, so anyone who is grieving gets given a copy as soon as they have encountered loss. They even write a personal message to the bereaved family in each book.

I would love people to do this with *Beyond Goodbye*. Maybe you feel you would like to be part of supporting others through grief and perhaps you could consider doing this?

For more information, email:
legacy@beyondgoodbye.org

About the Author

Zoë Clark-Coates BCAh is an award-winning charity CEO, business leader, counsellor, conference speaker, journalist, author and TV show host. For over 20 years she has been a trailblazer within PR, events and the media.

Following the loss of five babies, she co-founded the charity the Mariposa Trust (widely known by the name of its primary division, sayinggoodbye.org) with her husband Andy, enabling her to use her training as a counsellor on a daily basis.

As an innovative leader, she has steered the charity to become a leading support organisation in the UK and globally, providing support that reaches over 50,000 people each week.

As a gifted communicator, she has earned the respect of politicians, the government and many high-profile celebrities and influencers. Zoë's skill as a writer prompted Arianna Huffington to invite her to start writing for the *Huffington Post*, which created the perfect platform to reach a new audience and started her writing career. *Beyond Goodbye* is her third book on grief and loss. Her first book *Saying Goodbye* was an Amazon best seller, and her second book *The Baby Loss Guide* has been met with equal success and acclaim.

She has her own TV talk show called *Soul Tears*, where she interviews celebrities and people of note about their journeys through loss. She is also a trusted expert and media commentator for many other programmes on the BBC, ITV and Channel 5.

Zoë was appointed by the Secretary of State for Health as co-chair of the National Pregnancy Loss Review. As co-chair, she is responsible for advising the government and Department of Health on how better support and clinical care can be offered.